Advance Praise

"It is obvious that Jan has done extensive research in building practical tools to help patients, as well as health-care professionals, choose a well-defined path to good health. I support her approach and know readers will find her ideas invaluable. Our Texas roots steer us towards helping people. It is my hope that Jan's book will help others seamlessly weave the anti-inflammatory lifestyle into their busy lives."

—Barbara Bush, First Lady of the United States, 1989–1993

"I have spent years working with executives and associates who have entrepreneurial can-do spirits. It is clear to me these traits are strongest when individuals have done what it takes to maximize their health. Jan's book captures precise, logical, and useful tools all of us can use to improve our health and well-being. I recommend Jan's book and suggest others experience her ideas by applying them to their wellness plan. I do!"

—Ed Whitacre, Chairman Emeritus, AT&T
Former Chairman & CEO, General Motors Company

"Sleep is fuel for the brain, and without adequate rest the body's immune system is vulnerable to a high risk of hypertension, type 2 diabetes, obesity, Alzheimer's disease, and cancer, as well as a decrement in cognitive processing. Of all the nutrition and exercise books I'm familiar with, none until now have paid significant attention to the key role of sleep. Unfortunately, sleep is regarded by most people as a luxury rather than a necessity. But nutritionist, health educator, and author, Jan Tilley, is NOT asleep at the switch! *Eat Well to Be Well* is an incredibly well-written, concise, and scientifically based guide that reveals easy-to-follow tips on nutrition, exercise, stress reduction, and sleep. Logical and practical, Jan's book will convince you to adopt a lifestyle for guaranteed wellness and longevity."

—Dr. James B. Maas, Former Professor, Department Chair of Psychology,
and Stephen H. Weiss Presidential Fellow at Cornell University,
and Author of *Sleep for Success!* and *Sleep to Win!*

"Many Wells Fargo Advisor associates and clients know and love Jan for her passionate, engaging presentation style. She's worked with us for years helping to share practical wellness information at corporate and client events. I eagerly recommend *Eat Well to Be Well*, which beautifully defines how following a healthy, balanced lifestyle can be powerful medicine in helping us take charge of our health and well-being. Congratulations, Jan!"

—Keith Vanderveen, Regional President, Wells Fargo Advisors

"As a neurologist specializing in multiple sclerosis, I fully understand the powerful healing connection food, sleep, stress, and exercise can have on the journey to fight chronic disease. Jan understands and articulates how to focus on these areas as part of effective treatment and management. I am delighted to recommend her work."

—Dr. Ann Bass, Neurology Center of San Antonio

"Jan's new book is a dynamic compilation of scientific research and practical tools to equip fast-paced individuals to improve their health and wellness. The same vivacious spirit I see when Jan is speaking resonates in *Eat Well to Be Well*, inspiring readers to believe good health is possible and providing actionable steps to create a healthy, balanced lifestyle."

—Dr. Scott Livingston, EdD, MBA, Author of
7 Secrets of an Emotionally Intelligent Coach

"We can all realize improved energy, productivity, and focus if we determine to find our personal path to wellness. Jan's book is a creative tool kit for why and how to enjoy a healthier, happier life. I have personally experienced renewed energy in my own life since committing to these healthy changes. Let me encourage you to invest in yourself; you won't be disappointed. Thank you, Jan!"

—Diane Dalton Warren, Founder of Bounceology
and Former SVP of Clear Channel Worldwide

JAN TILLEY, MS RDN LD

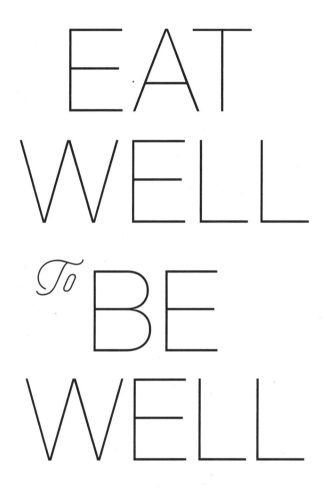

EAT WELL

To BE WELL

LIVING YOUR BEST LIFE THROUGH
the POWER *of* ANTI-INFLAMMATORY FOOD

BOOK THREE OF THE LIVE WELL TO BE WELL SERIES

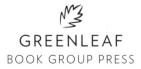

GREENLEAF
BOOK GROUP PRESS

Published by Greenleaf Book Group Press
Austin, Texas
www.gbgpress.com

Distributed by Greenleaf Book Group

For ordering information or special discounts for bulk purchases, please contact Greenleaf Book Group at PO Box 91869, Austin, TX 78709, 512.891.6100.

Design and composition by Greenleaf Book Group
Cover design by Greenleaf Book Group
Cover images: ©Shutterstock.com/Serg64, ©istock.com/Halfpoint
Recipe photos by Joe Houde—Houde Studio

Publisher's Cataloging-in-Publication Data is available.

ISBN: 978-1-62634-266-8

TreeNeutral®

Printed in Canada on acid-free paper

15 16 17 18 19 20   10 9 8 7 6 5 4 3 2 1

First Edition

Other Edition(s):
eBook ISBN: 978-1-62634-267-5

Whether your goal is to do whatever it takes to prevent chronic inflammation and avoid chronic disease, or if you are already battling against disease that has been brought on by inflammation, I want you to know that good health is possible. It takes time, effort, dedication, and determination, but the reward of a long, healthy, happy life is SO worth your investment! —Jan Tilley

Contents

Foreword

America is heading for a health crisis. In the opinion of many, we are already there, and the rest of the world is not far behind. It is projected that chronic inflammatory diseases—including heart disease, cancer, Alzheimer's, diabetes, and obesity, among others—will stress our healthcare system to its breaking point in the next ten to fifteen years. In *Eat Well to Be Well: Living Your Best Life through the Power of Anti-Inflammatory Food*, Jan Tilley expertly summarizes the pending risks to our health stemming from chronic inflammation. Arguing that the commonplace diet has become completely unbalanced, she provides a commonsense approach to reconstructing a lifestyle that brings balance into our system. Among these precepts are using foods as medicines, maintaining a healthy weight, and managing stress.

Eat Well to Be Well: Living Your Best Life through the Power of Anti-Inflammatory Food starts with Tilley's personal experience in her clinical dietary practice, observing firsthand the impact of out-of-control inflammation on her clients. From these experiences, she has constructed a useful guide to creating your own Anti-Inflammatory Plan, in the hopes of empowering all of us to bring balance back into our lives as one strategy to offset the coming tidal wave of chronic inflammatory diseases.

This book will be a valuable asset for years to come and should be read by all seeing their doctor in the hopes of avoiding or reducing the severity of these formidable diseases.

Michael J. Wargovich, Ph.D.
Professor of Molecular Medicine
Cancer Center Council Distinguished Chair in Oncology
UT Regents Health Research Scholar
Department of Molecular Medicine
University of Texas Health Sciences Center at San Antonio

Acknowledgments

I would like to thank the following amazing team of people who surrounded me as I wrote *Eat Well to Be Well* and who moved mountains to help make this book a reality.

First of all, my husband, Bruce, who has supported and encouraged me every step of the way—from allowing me countless hours of uninterrupted writing solitude on the back patio to giving vision and insight on making the manuscript into a book that will reach, teach, and inspire readers to do whatever it takes to pursue health.

My clients who inspire me daily! It is my privilege to witness your determination to chase after health in spite of obstacles that would seem overwhelming to most. Thank you for allowing me to be a part of your health journey.

Mary Jane, my practice manager, chief of staff, and dear friend, who has worked tirelessly to facilitate all aspects of getting this book to print. She believes with her whole heart that the work we do saves lives by helping people take charge of their health. Her faith in me and in our work motivates me to be my very best every day.

Diane Warren, my business strategist and consultant extraordinaire, who has pushed me to reach for goals beyond my wildest expectations. Her ability to bounce into a project, determine a strategic plan for tackling it, then roll up her sleeves and help make it a reality is unmatched by anyone anywhere.

To Larry Hoberman, Dr. James Maas, and Dr. Michael Wargovich for their contribution as subject matter experts to the content of *Eat Well to Be Well*. Because of their willingness to share their knowledge and expertise, this book has become a powerful source of the most current information on managing chronic disease.

Mary Anne Toepperwein, who with her past experience as Educational Development Specialist, Department of Medicine, University of Texas Health Science Center at San Antonio, Texas, was a godsend to me. She reviewed mounds of studies to help me identify the most credible anti-inflammatory research. She eagerly did whatever else I needed to finalize references, proof-read chapters, and so much more.

Nicki Ortiz, who painstakingly analyzed each recipe in this book while taking time to check and recheck for nutritional accuracy. Her attention to detail is unparalleled and greatly appreciated!

My mom, Ganelle Pearce Hampton, who spent countless hours proofing. My publisher said it was one of the cleanest manuscripts they'd ever seen when they got it!

Joe and Carole Houde, who gave us a fabulous weekend of food styling and photography. It was a weekend of cooking none of us will soon forget! Your professionalism, creativity, and expertise were paramount to creating this beautiful book! Charlene Lowe, my neighbor and friend, who graciously came to help as my sous chef.

Mary Kaye Sawyer-Morse, who made her passion for living the anti-inflammatory lifestyle contagious! She helped create many of the book's practical tools and was encouraging and instrumental in getting this book to print.

My clinical team of registered dietitians, Krista Neugebauer, Sam Lopez, Libby Higham, and Daniel Guerra, who were willing to pick up the slack in our JTA clinic to allow me time to write, create, and dream. You've been the bedrock upon which this book was built. Thank you all!

Greenleaf Book Group, who provided leadership and direction in editing, design, and distribution. I appreciate all you've done to help *Eat Well to Be Well* become a reality!

And last but not least, thank you to all of you—our readers—who are actively searching for your path to wellness. I pray this book will contain the practical tools you need to conquer chronic disease and maximize your health.

What is Inflammation?

What do an ant bite, a splinter, and the flu virus all have in common? All represent examples of *acute inflammation*; the kind of inflammation that calls on our body's immune system to respond swiftly to repair damage and shuts down just as quickly once the healing is complete. Very efficient! On the other hand, what do high-fat diets, sugary treats, poor sleep habits, repeated stress, and lack of exercise have in common? Each of these cause harm to our body gradually over a longer period of time. Our immune system fights to repair the problem, but in this case it reacts more slowly and does not know when to stop. This scenario, where our body mistakenly identifies healthy tissues as harmful pathogens, is known as *chronic inflammation*.

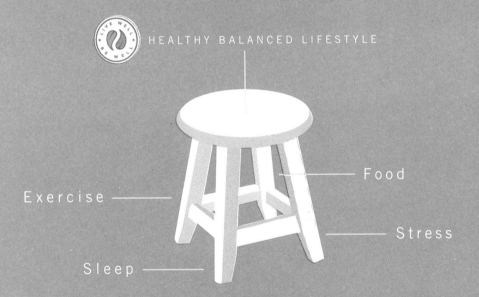

HEALTHY BALANCED LIFESTYLE

Food

Exercise

Stress

Sleep

Introduction

Food is medicine—and it has an amazing power to
heal, repair, and maximize the human potential!

After more than twenty years as a registered dietitian coaching
others to take charge of their health, I am more convinced than
ever of the vital role that nutrition, exercise, sleep, and stress
management play in promoting health. I like to refer to these key components as the four-legged stool of a balanced, healthy lifestyle. In my practice,
I have been privileged to see the powerful transformation that occurs when
patients commit to making healthy changes in the way they fuel, move, and
rest their bodies.

Years of study and observation as a clinician have led me to realize that
one of the best tools we have to maximize health and reverse chronic disease is to reduce the chronic inflammation in our bodies. While the path to
decreasing inflammation is not rocket science, it is a matter of redefining the
food, fitness, and lifestyle choices we make.

I've chosen to write this book to give you science-based facts, practical tools, and deliciously simple recipes to guide you toward health. I passionately believe that by increasing anti-inflammatory foods and decreasing pro-inflammatory foods in our diet, we can stave off and even reverse many of the horrible chronic disease processes we see as we age.

One of the most exciting facts I have learned from studying and practicing the anti-inflammatory diet is that it can be effective even if you cannot follow it perfectly—making it practical for all of us! There is, however, a direct correlation between how stringently we follow the anti-inflammatory (AI) lifestyle and the resulting reversal of chronic disease.

In the pages that follow, you will find a well-defined path to help you take charge of your health. From the first chapter, I will define the anti-inflammatory lifestyle and will guide you to make small but significant changes to incorporate it into your life. It is my sincere hope that you will take this opportunity to discover for yourself the power you have to create a healthier, happier you.

My goal in writing *Eat Well to Be Well* is to give you a glimpse into the benefits of the Anti-Inflammatory (AI) lifestyle and give you the practical tools you will need to apply it to your life. I hope my words and suggestions will stir within you the desire to do whatever it takes to pursue good health.

Chapter 1

Understanding Inflammation

Centuries ago Hippocrates, the Father of Modern Medicine, said, "Let food be thy medicine and medicine thy food." We have known for a very long time that food is medicine and that it has the amazing power to heal, repair, and maximize the human potential!

I am passionate about the impact healthy choices can have in our lives. Whether you are seeking to follow an anti-inflammatory lifestyle to live the healthiest, best life possible, or you are seeking a holistic approach to managing chronic disease, it is my goal to give you tools you need to take charge of your health.

I see anti-inflammatory living as being a four-legged stool comprised of balanced nutrition, moderate exercise, managed stress, and high-quality sleep. Each of these will be discussed at length in this book, giving you practical, actionable steps to help you achieve optimum health and well-being.

For many, aging may mean settling for aches, pains, and physical limitations, writing them off as simply a reality of aging. The remedy of choice is often to add a host of medications to help manage symptoms and pain. This is not the only solution! Growing older does not have to mean growing sicker! We all have the choice to make lifestyle decisions to do everything within our control to stave off chronic disease. I am not suggesting that a healthy lifestyle will allow you to avoid all disease, but I am saying that healthy choices give you a real fighting chance to live a healthy, strong, vibrant life well into old age. I believe better health is possible for all of us, and it is my hope that by the time you finish reading this book you will believe it, too!

"Let food be thy medicine and medicine thy food."

To appreciate the importance of anti-inflammatory living, it is important to fully understand inflammation and the effects it can have on our body. I see the impact of inflammation demonstrated over and over again in the lives of our patients. At JTA Wellness (JTA) we care for people every day in our clinic who are broken and suffering with chronic disease, with obesity, and with physical bodies that are breaking down well before their time.

What is Inflammation?

What do an ant bite, a splinter, and the flu virus all have in common? All represent examples of *acute inflammation*; the kind of inflammation that calls on our body's immune system to respond swiftly to repair damage and to shut down just as quickly once the healing is complete. Very efficient! On the other hand, what do high-fat diets, sugary treats, poor sleep habits, repeated stress, and lack of exercise have in common? Each of these causes harm to our body gradually over a longer period of time. Our immune system fights to repair the problem, but in these cases it reacts more slowly and does not know when to stop. This scenario, where our body mistakenly identifies healthy tissues as harmful pathogens, is known as *chronic inflammation*. There is a growing body of evidence that leads us to believe that chronic inflammation is responsible for many of the chronic diseases we see as we age, including type 2 diabetes, cardiovascular disease, arthritis, cognitive decline, and some types of cancer.

Symptoms associated with chronic inflammation can range from no symptoms at all to things like joint pain/arthritis; fatigue; bloating; abdominal pain; skin rashes; elevated cholesterol, triglyceride, and glucose levels; and cognitive decline. If chronic inflammation is left untreated, this diagram shows the diseases that can result:

> Healthy choices give you a real fighting chance to live a healthy, strong, vibrant life well into old age.

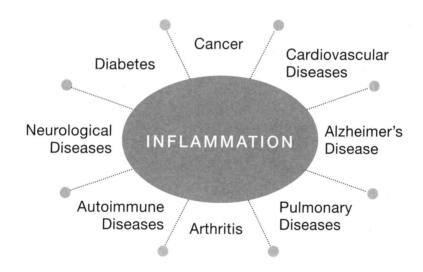

Often chronic inflammation creeps up so slowly that we simply attribute the aches and pains we are experiencing to the inevitable aging process. Or we are diagnosed with a chronic disease and think "Ugh, just my luck, bad genetics!" Rather than assume fate has dealt us a low blow, let's make sure we have a clear definition of what it means to be healthy—regardless of our age.

There are numerous factors that can contribute to chronic inflammation. During the course of this book, we will be discussing how to avoid pro-inflammatory factors and how to adopt more anti-inflammatory behaviors. There are a variety of things that promote inflammation, including

- Obesity—by far the biggest risk factor when it comes to chronic inflammation!
- Stress
- Smoking (first- and secondhand smoke)
- Sugar
- Saturated and Trans Fats
- Highly Processed Foods
- Poor or Inadequate Sleep
- Sedentary Lifestyle or Excessive Exercise

If exposed long enough to factors that promote inflammation, we will likely develop symptoms that ultimately lead to chronic disease. To combat chronic inflammation, we must take a look at behaviors that prevent it, such as

- Eating More Anti-inflammatory Foods
- Maintaining a Healthy Weight
- Engaging in Moderate Exercise
- Practicing Stress Management
- Getting Adequate High-Quality Sleep

The following diagram is a simple depiction of foods that are harmful, pro-inflammatory choices versus healthy, anti-inflammatory foods that will help fight against chronic inflammation. In upcoming chapters we will delve deeper into specific foods that provide the greatest AI benefit.

Foods to Choose/Foods to Avoid

Now that we have defined chronic inflammation and identified behavioral changes we can make to prevent or reverse its effects, let's take a look at defining health. Some would laugh and say, "Isn't health the absence of disease?" I believe good health is so much more!

Pro-Inflammatory Foods (Eliminate or Limit in Diet)

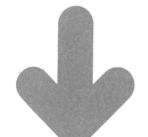

- Trans fats/partially hydrogenated fats
- Saturated fats and omega-6 fatty acids (for example, corn oil, many salad dressings, and snack foods)
- Sugar
- White breads, pastas, pastries
- Whole-fat dairy
- Processed meats

Anti-Inflammatory Foods (Increase in Diet)

- Healthy fats: avocado, olives, and extra-virgin olive oil
- Healthy protein: wild-caught fish, lean meat, beans, and nuts
- Complex carbohydrates: quinoa, brown rice, sweet potatoes, winter squash
- Vegetables: good choices include dark green leafy vegetables, broccoli, cauliflower, bok choy, carrots, radishes, beets
- Fruits: good choices include apples, pears, berries, grapes, melons, mangoes, kiwi

Chapter 2

Healthy Looks So Good on You!

Healthy is not something that magically happens to us. It is something we must intentionally pursue. It is something we must fight for. Choosing healthy behaviors has the power to transform your appearance, your energy, and your LIFE!

Healthy is a look, an aura of well-being, a vibrant skin tone, a personal countenance that you can't fake—it can't be created as a facade. It can only appear as a result of building health from the inside out.

Have you taken a good long look in the mirror? What do you see?

Baggy Eyes or Bright Eyes

Drawn Mouth or Dazzling Smile

Sallow Complexion or Rosy Cheeks

Puffy Face or Radiant Skin

Fatigue or Energy

Our physical appearance is a visible barometer of our state of health. If you look in the mirror and don't see that youthful sparkle you once had, perhaps it is time to reevaluate your health status. Read on and you will discover small but significant changes you can make that will help promote your healthy glow once again!

• • •

In my opinion, nothing communicates better than a personal story. I have asked a few of my clients for permission to share their stories with you so you can witness what a difference embracing a healthy lifestyle has made in their lives.

The first patient I'd like to introduce you to is Kathy. She arrived at my office with a myriad of health complications and weight issues she had been dealing with for years. Now, two years later, she has done a remarkable job of taking charge of her choices and getting her life back.

When I first met Kathy, she was a very strong personality with her own ideas of how our sessions were going to go. She comes by that honestly as she is the retired President/CEO of a large organization. She and her delightfully supportive husband are now retired and splitting their time between the Texas Hill Country and the state of Oregon when Texas gets too hot!

Initially, Kathy was seeking a weight-loss solution that allowed her to continue in her current indulgent lifestyle. My suggestion to limit her portion size on food and wine and include more exercise was met with resistance. However, she made a couple of changes, saw some success, and increased her energy. This encouraged her to make still more changes, and now she is an amazing example of how to recreate yourself to enjoy the

> Our physical appearance is a visible barometer of our state of health.

second half of life! When I asked Kathy to give me her thoughts on how she made the transition from chronic disease to wellness, she wrote these very insightful comments for me. I hope you will find inspiration and encouragement through her story.

"At my first meeting with Jan I felt like we were having a shared conversation, not a lecture. Jan 'got me' and I felt like she was pulling for my success as much as I was. Initially the concept of healthy living inside and out was not what I wanted to hear about—I just wanted a good diet plan. Having failed at every diet out there, I really never expected this plan to actually work! I didn't want details; just a quick fix! I couldn't get Jan to give in. As we kept talking, I acknowledged other health issues besides my weight that I had written off to job stress and just getting older, which for me translated to 'I can't do anything about this.'

"Nutrition counseling at JTA offered me REAL accountability. I have a long history of being an 'annual dieter.' Each year I told myself that this was the year I was going to lose weight. I would select a date to start and two weeks later I was already building up the list of reasons this diet was probably not going to work. The only people who knew I was even trying were family members who never expected me to stick with it anyway. Real accountability is when you tell your closest friends, those you respect the most, and the ones who will be truly disappointed if you fail again. If you are embarrassed about quitting, you have told the right people. With Jan's help I was able to be transparent enough to admit I was trying to get healthy.

"For years my favorite line was to tell people I was born a size 14 and it has been all uphill from there. I seriously have a pair of black slacks in every full and half size ever made because this was going to be the year the weight came off. No more! Now every time I drop a size I get rid of those clothes—no going back to the old me!

"Perhaps the most sobering realization I've had on this journey to health is that with all my professional accomplishments, I had not found the willpower and courage to fight for me. With Jan's direction and the love and support of my family and friends, I've been able to prove to myself that I could be the person I always knew I was deep inside. I have found the courage to believe in myself!

"In addition to motivating me to meet my weight-loss goals, Jan taught me how to use food and exercise to battle my other chronic health issues including high cholesterol, prediabetes, and high blood pressure. Her expertise in reviewing my lab values helped encourage me to stay the course even when the scale was not moving as fast as I thought it should! I had been unaware of the high level of medical expertise I would be getting at JTA. Together, we did it—I've lost 54 pounds and my lab results are all within normal range.

"The best thing about the new me is that I have the energy, stamina, and good health to enjoy my retirement years. I've had to moderate my portions and find physical activities I enjoy, but that has been a very small price to pay for the amazing energetic life I've discovered. I can honestly say now that I LOVE my life!"

The message I want you to glean from Kathy's journey back to health is this—our bodies are wonderfully resilient and the health that we can regain from staying focused on a few small but significant changes is nothing short of miraculous! Food really does have the power to heal!

There is no substitute for the authentic beauty that being healthy on the inside brings to the outside!

• • •

Describe your health vision. What does good health look like to you? _____

_____

_____

_____

What is your biggest motivator to make a lifestyle change? _____

_____

_____

_____

What changes do you need to make to pursue health? _____

_____

_____

_____

Chapter 3

Chronic Inflammation and Your Gut

We know that good health creates an outward vitality that is easy to identify, but there is a LOT going on inside our body as well. Our intestinal tract is constantly bombarded with potentially harmful toxins and organisms we ingest in our diet. The intestinal immune system is constantly monitoring for suspicious pathogenic products and harmful bugs. As a consequence, our gut can be both a target and an instigator of acute and chronic inflammation.

As a Target

When your gut is the target of an inflammatory attack, inflammatory bowel disease (IBD) can result. Ulcerative Colitis and Crohn's disease are two major types of IBD that have active periods when inflammation is high, followed by inactive times when inflammation is low. The cause of IBD is typically some

> By eating a healthy diet, managing stress, and avoiding certain medications, it is possible to increase helpful bacteria and reduce gut inflammation.

combination of genes, environment, and the immune system coming together to trigger bowel disease. Generally, people with IBD have a relative with the same disorder. There is a genetic tendency for the immune system in people with IBD to mount full-blown inflammatory attacks on harmless bacteria commonly found in their intestinal tract. This genetic tendency is related to a flaw in how the immune system recognizes friendly and harmful bacteria. By eating a healthy diet, managing stress, and avoiding certain medications, it is possible to increase helpful bacteria and reduce gut inflammation. If left unmanaged, IBD can lead to arthritis; cardiovascular, skin, liver, and kidney disease; bone loss; anemia; and malnutrition. Controlling chronic inflammation to prevent flare-ups is a major goal in IBD.

Irritable Bowel Syndrome (IBS) is often confused with IBD, but the two are very different. We will discuss IBS in more depth later in this chapter.

As an Instigator

Evidence is mounting about the role our gut plays as an instigator of chronic inflammation and related autoimmune disease. Increased attention from researchers on the source of chronic inflammation in our bodies has revealed a relatively new culprit known as leaky gut. It appears that our lifestyle choices may trigger this condition, which is now a known contributor to a wide number of autoimmune health concerns from arthritis to multiple sclerosis. Research is beginning to identify important steps you can take to repair leaky gut and create a healthy microbiome, which may further empower your body to fight off chronic inflammation.

What Is Leaky Gut?

To help you better understand what leaky gut means, it may help to provide a visual. Imagine a newly built brick wall with mortar tightly filling the gaps between bricks so completely there's no space for anything to seep through. Now, visualize that same wall a decade later, poorly maintained, with bricks shifting and starting to crumble as the mortar begins to lose its ability to hold the wall together. In fact, if you look closely, you can see spaces between bricks where none existed before.

Using that imaginary wall as an example, think of the bricks as protective cells and the mortar as tight junctions between cells in the lining of your gut. In this case, the tight junctions are created by secreted proteins, such as zonulin, which act to reinforce the lining, making it impermeable to all but the most vital substances necessary to maintain good health.

Health problems may arise when those tight junctions become compromised and permeable, allowing unintended substances, like undigested food and toxic waste products, bacteria, and viruses, to "leak" through your vulnerable gut lining and into your bloodstream. These toxic invaders circulate throughout the body, forcing your body's immune system to react. This inflammation can result in a wide range of symptoms—from stomach cramps, food sensitivities, and fatigue to headaches and aching joints.

What Triggers Leaky Gut?

Some factors that can damage the intestinal barrier and lead to leaky gut include

- Unhealthy Food Choices (such as highly refined carbohydrates)
- Foods to Which You Are Allergic

In addition to these factors, there are two fascinating areas of research into the mechanism that may trigger leaky gut.

1. Zonulin, the protein we've noted that helps prevent tight junctions from becoming too porous, has been the target of a number of studies. It now appears that too much zonulin may contribute to a weakening of proteins along the lining of the gut, resulting in more intestinal permeability, i.e., leaky gut. In a clinical trial involving celiac patients exposed to gluten, scientists calculated a 70 percent increase in intestinal permeability along with elevated levels of zonulin.

2. As research progresses, another possible player in the leaky gut saga has emerged. Lipopolysaccharides (LPS) are endotoxins that may be released either as normal secretions or after damage to the cell wall. The release of LPS via the leaky gut into the bloodstream signals a worsening of inflammation. How serious is this increase in LPS? Some health experts claim physicians may successfully predict the life expectancy of heart attack patients in ICUs based solely on LPS levels in their blood.

- Excessive Intake of Alcohol and Caffeine
- Poor Stress Management
- Overuse of Antibiotics
- Overgrowth of Harmful Bacteria in the Gut

Are Processed Foods the Enemy?

Unfortunately, our busy lifestyles can often play havoc with our quest for health. Our fast food eating habits may be helping to crumble the internal brick wall that protects our bodies from harm. Eating a diet rich in plant-based whole foods, with plenty of non-soluble dietary fiber, keeps that tight red brick wall intact, preventing the gut wall from becoming porous and leaky.

What Can Be Done to Build a Healthier Gut?

The health of our gut actually begins at birth. In utero, we are swimming around in amniotic fluid, not yet using our intestines. At birth, we travel through the vaginal canal and ingest our mother's healthy intestinal bacteria. These bacteria are crucial in signaling the normal development of the intestinal lining and immune system (70 percent of our immune system is in the intestines). Newborns feed on breast milk, which contains resistant starches. The bacteria are able to break down or ferment the resistant starches in breast milk that are not digested by the small intestines. These starches arrive intact at the colon, where the bacteria ferment the starches to produce short chain fatty acids (SCFA) called butyrate, acetate, and propionate. The SCFA provide nourishment for the colon lining cells and signal the maturation of the intestinal lining cells and immune system.

The health of our gut actually begins at birth.

Starting out at birth with a healthy gut was obviously something out of our control, but there are steps we can take now to help build healthier intestines. Daily intake of prebiotics (resistant starches) has been found to be an important dietary aid in maintaining healthy intestinal bacteria. Prebiotics contain starches that cannot be digested by our intestinal enzymes, so they escape to the colon. Bacteria in the colon ferment the starches producing the important SCFA, and the starches provide nourishment for these bacteria, so they can flourish.

Adding healthy, anti-inflammatory foods containing high amounts of prebiotics and probiotics from natural food sources to our diet are all key to healing leaky gut syndrome and promoting the growth of healthy bacteria in the intestines. Such foods include

- leeks, asparagus, artichokes, garlic, onions, wheat, oats, soybeans, bananas, artichokes, and blueberries
- Greek yogurt and kefir
- fermented plant-based foods such as sauerkraut
- broccoli and other cruciferous vegetables

For a complete listing of healthy prebiotic and probiotic foods, visit our website at www.jtawellness.com/probioticfoods.

Probiotic supplements are also often recommended to help restore friendly gut bacteria. It is now commonplace to see probiotics recommended to heal a damaged gut lining to prevent it from leaking. Our understanding of how to manipulate our gut microbiota is still in the early stages, and clearly more high-quality studies are needed to define the best protocol for probiotic use. The best advice is to follow the guidance of your physician when deciding to use a probiotic supplement. Most will recommend a supplement that contains at least ten billion bacteria containing both *Lactobacillus* and *Bifidobacterium* strains. Studies have shown these two bacteria are important in reducing intestinal inflammation and enhancing production of the important short chain fatty acids. Some probiotics also contain a prebiotic, which, as you now know, helps to maintain the healthy intestinal bacteria.

Is There a Connection Between IBS, Leaky Gut, and FODMAP Foods?

There is another phenomenon that may play a part in the instigation of IBS and leaky gut. These are high FODMAP foods.

What is FODMAP?

While discussing FODMAP is like opening a giant can of worms, I feel it is a very important topic to discuss in a chapter about chronic inflammation and your gut. Many gastroenterologists today are prescribing a low FODMAP diet to help manage IBS. FODMAP is an acronym referring to Fermentable Oligo-saccharides, Disaccharides, Monosaccharides, and Polyols, and can be defined as a group of fermentable short chain carbohydrates that some people have difficulty digesting. These short chain carbohydrates may sit in the gut, ferment, and cause many of the symptoms associated with IBS such as gas, bloating, pain, and intermittent constipation and diarrhea. IBS is often confused with Inflammatory Bowel Disease (IBD), but the two are very different. IBS is a functional disorder characterized by abdominal discomfort, diarrhea or constipation, or alternating between the two. It is likely caused by the way the brain and gut interact, causing irregular patterns of muscle contractions in the intestines.

Recent compelling research from Monash University in Melbourne, Australia, indicates that consumption of high FODMAP foods may instigate IBS symptoms in those incapable of digesting these short chain carbohydrates. It is important to note that a low FODMAP diet eliminates all FODMAP foods for a period of six to eight weeks. The process should be overseen by a dietitian, trained in working with IBS patients, who will help the client reintroduce foods back into their diet one at a time. The goal would be to ultimately end up with only a handful of foods that may need to be completely eliminated for life.

 To find a more complete discussion of the FODMAP diet, visit our website at www.jtawellness.com/FODMAP

To give you an idea of how powerful FODMAP can be, let me share Janis's story with you. She is a delightful patient I recently counseled who was president of a large political organization, very active in her church, and had many other family and social obligations. She complained of experiencing an urgency to run to the bathroom from five to ten times a day. Her fear of needing to be close to a bathroom was interfering with her life. She had been recently diagnosed with IBS, and her physician sent her to me to help teach her the FODMAP diet. Within days of eliminating all FODMAP foods, she was drastically improved, and within weeks she was completely back to normal and enjoying her very busy life. If the inability to digest high FODMAP foods is the cause of your IBS, the impact of eliminating these foods can be life-changing.

A few years ago, when I first began seeing referrals from physicians requesting instruction for their patients on a FODMAP diet, I have to admit I was skeptical about its efficacy. After years of working with it, I have seen a dramatic improvement in the lives of many of my patients and have become a proponent of using this diet.

It is clear that our gastrointestinal system is intricately linked to chronic inflammation. Research in this field is expanding rapidly and promises many new and exciting treatments for some of our most common and debilitating chronic diseases. The key to preventing inflammation in our gut is not a medicine cabinet full of prescriptions. It is found in the healing power of adopting a healthy anti-inflammatory lifestyle. In the chapters that follow, I will guide you through a step-by-step, practical approach to building a healthy body by balancing nutrition, enjoying moderate exercise, managing stress, and getting adequate good sleep.

This chapter was written in cooperation with Dr. Lawrence J. Hoberman. He has spent more than forty years practicing medicine and is board certified in both Internal Medicine (1972) and Gastroenterology (1975). He is currently in practice at Health by Design, located in San Antonio, Texas.

Chapter 4

Eat Well to Be Well

*I*n the first three chapters of this book we have reviewed inflammation, where it comes from, and the results than can occur if it is left unmanaged. Now that you have a good basic understanding of inflammation and have made it through a pretty hefty science chapter on intestinal health, the next few chapters will focus on what you can do to take charge of your health. We will take a look at the vital role that nutrition, exercise, sleep, and stress management play in promoting health. I like to refer to these key components as the four-legged stool of a balanced, healthy lifestyle. If these are the legs, we must know that the base of the stool that holds everything together is maintaining a healthy weight. When weight starts to creep up, inflammation and chronic health issues are close behind.

Nutrition, exercise, sleep, and stress management play vital roles in promoting health.

I would have to say that the most insidious condition I see as a clinician is obesity. On the surface it may look like simply a weight problem, but the reality

Obesity is an epidemic and is the **leading** worldwide public health problem. Weight loss is the key to reducing chronic inflammation and resulting pathologies (Fernandez-Sanchez et al.). While public health efforts have resulted in improved blood pressure, lowered smoking rates, and reduced cholesterol levels, epidemic obesity and type 2 diabetes have increased. Epidemic obesity is associated with alarming health problems. We know that reducing excess fat tissue, especially harmful belly fat, is key to preventing and or reversing chronic inflammation and resulting diseases (Mathieu, Lemieux, and Des).

Over the past two decades, new insights into the inner workings of fat tissue have changed our understanding. Fat tissue stores energy, but that is not all it does. We now know that when fat tissue increases, it becomes the largest endocrine organ in our bodies. How? There is a complex interaction with our immune system that causes chronic inflammation (Kim et al.). In fact, obesity can be considered a state of chronic inflammation that causes other areas of chronic inflammation in our bodies (Nathan).

is, obesity destroys health. A large majority of the patients we see in our practice are obese and are dealing with joint pain, pre- or full-blown diabetes, hypertension, high cholesterol, high triglycerides, accelerated aging, limitations in movement, and so much more. We know that obesity is a state of chronic inflammation that leads to chronic disease. If we can help clients decrease weight, they can begin to decrease inflammation and thus manage their disease. At JTA Wellness our approach in the initial appointment with obese clients is to help them lose 5 to 10 percent of their body weight. It is truly amazing how just a small amount of weight loss can significantly improve their blood sugar, blood pressure, and cholesterol numbers, bringing them back into a more normal range. While having your clothes fit a bit more loosely is a wonderful side benefit, the major focus of weight loss is to manage the chronic diseases that have surfaced secondary to obesity.

Weight loss isn't easy. You must passionately seek it and be willing to discipline yourself to achieve it. I have a saying I've used for years that says it best—"What are you willing to sacrifice for what you want to become?" There is always a cost associated with making a lifestyle change. It may be a sacrifice of time, money, sleep, or other resources, but choosing health will not just land in your lap. It always comes at a price. The good news is, the return on your investment will be a life free of many of the health complications associated with obesity. By losing weight, you are taking the most important step toward conquering chronic inflammation. Weight loss is the first step toward taking charge of your health to embrace the anti-inflammatory lifestyle.

Body Mass Index (BMI) & Waist Circumference (WC)

There are two tools I find most helpful in determining obesity and the risk for chronic disease. The first is body mass index (BMI), which is based on body weight and height. While BMI is not foolproof, it is a good guide to help determine a patient's goal weight and their caloric needs for weight loss. The goal is to have a BMI between 18 and 25. As we age, I like my clients to stay closer to a BMI in the upper range of normal so they have some padding in case they get sick and don't feel like eating for a few days.

BMI alone has limitations and can lead to the misclassification of certain individuals, such as those with increased muscle mass or the elderly. At JTA we use a combination of waist circumference and BMI to help determine a client's risk for disease. Waist circumference is particularly useful for individuals with a BMI of 25-34.

A high waist circumference or a greater level of abdominal fat is associated with an increased risk for type 2 diabetes, high cholesterol, high blood pressure, and heart disease. According to the United States Department of Health and Human Services (HHS) the following individuals are at increased risk for developing chronic diseases:

> While BMI is not foolproof, it is a good guide to help determine a patient's goal weight and their caloric needs for weight loss.

- Women with a waist circumference of more than 35 inches
- Men with a waist circumference of more than 40 inches

 To determine your BMI and find instructions for how to properly measure for waist circumference visit our website at www.jtawellness.com/BMIcalculator. To determine your calorie needs for weight management; and obtain a personalized plan to help you meet your goals, visit our website to join our membership program at www.jtawellness.com/lifestylemanagementprogram.

The anti-inflammatory lifestyle is not a quick-fix weight loss plan, but most overweight people who adopt this lifestyle will lose weight and inches. As we take a look at how to eat well to be well, we are not only fighting obesity; we are doing everything possible to balance our health to successfully battle inflammation.

To build the healthiest AI eating plan, there are foods to choose more often and foods to eliminate in order to fight chronic disease. To help you navigate using the best science-based information, we will identify foods, herbs, and spices that can be used to dramatically increase the absorption and effectiveness of anti-inflammatory foods.

There are two major categories of food that are important to discuss when building an anti-inflammatory eating plan.

1. Foods to Avoid: Pro-inflammatory foods that promote chronic inflammation in our bodies such as sugar, highly processed foods, and saturated fats.

2. Foods to Choose: Anti-inflammatory foods such as fruits, vegetables, whole grains, and lean proteins that help decrease chronic inflammation by protecting cells and bolstering immune function.

Anti-Inflammatory & Pro-Inflammatory Foods

Carbohydrates

Anti-Inflammatory:

- Fruits
- Vegetables
- Whole grains such as quinoa, whole wheat, steel-cut oats
- Low-fat dairy

Pro-Inflammatory:

- Sugar and other sweeteners such as high fructose corn syrup
- Processed flour and its by-products such as white bread, pasta, crackers, desserts made from sugar and processed flour such as cakes, cookies, pies
- Processed grains such as white rice, refined cereals
- Full-fat dairy

Proteins

Anti-Inflammatory:

- Fish—especially those rich in omega-3 fats like salmon, tuna, and lake trout
- Chicken—especially white meat without the skin
- Lean pork and beef trimmed of all visible fat
- Vegetarian protein sources such as lentils, soy, and legumes
- Low-fat cheese
- Eggs
- Nuts and nut butters

Pro-Inflammatory:

- Processed meat such as hot dogs, bologna, salami
- High fat meats such as marbled beef, sausage, bacon
- Full-fat cheese

Fats

Anti-Inflammatory:

- Avocado
- Olive or canola oil (expeller-pressed canola is best)
- Nuts and nut butters
- Ground flaxseed, chia seed, pumpkin, sunflower, and sesame seeds

Pro-Inflammatory:

- Saturated fats such as shortening, butter, cream
- Trans fats (can be found in some commercial baked goods and movie popcorn)
- Omega-6 oils such as corn and vegetable oil
- Poultry skin and meat fat

The Basics

To help you determine which foods are your best choices, I've created a list by nutrient group for you. Build your food choices from the anti-inflammatory list and avoid foods from the pro-inflammatory list.

Polyphenols

Of all the anti-inflammatory substances being studied, I find the research on polyphenols to be fascinating. I promise not to go too "science nerd" on you, but take a look at this: Polyphenols (such as ellagic acid and resveratrol) may help prevent cancer formation, prevent inflammation, and work as antioxidants. Some examples of foods containing polyphenols are green tea, grapes, wine, berries, citrus fruits, apples, whole grains, and peanuts. The health effects of polyphenols depend upon the amount consumed and their bioavailability.

Not all polyphenols are absorbed with equal efficacy. They are extensively metabolized by intestinal and liver enzymes and by the normal intestinal microbes (microflora).

Numerous factors can affect the polyphenol content of plants, including ripeness at the time of harvest, processing, and storage. Environmental factors such as soil, sun exposure, and rainfall can also have a major effect on a plant's polyphenol content. Agronomic factors such as whether plants were grown in greenhouses or fields and amount of yield per tree can also play a role in polyphenol content.

Here are just a few interesting examples of how varied polyphenol levels can be within the same variety of produce.

- Because the solid parts of citrus fruit, particularly the white spongy portion (albedo) and the membranes separating the segments, have a very high polyphenol content, the whole fruit may contain up to five times as much as a glass of orange juice. This is why we say "Eat your fruit, don't drink it!"

- In leafy vegetables such as lettuce and cabbage, the concentration is as much as ten times higher in the green outer leaves as in the inner light-colored leaves.

- Marked differences in concentration exist between pieces of fruit on the same tree and even between different sides of a single piece of fruit, depending on exposure to sunlight.

- Cherry tomatoes typically have a higher polyphenol content than standard tomatoes, because they have higher proportions of skin and outer surface exposed to sunlight than larger tomatoes.

Storage and cooking technique are two additional things that can have a major effect on the concentration of polyphenols. Storage can directly affect the polyphenol content of fruits and vegetables due to the easy oxidation of polyphenols. Once produce is harvested, it begins to lose key nutrients (such as polyphenols) during transport and storage. This is one of the biggest reasons why it is important to buy local produce when possible so that the time between harvest and purchase is kept to a minimum. Cooking technique can also play a big role in polyphenol concentration. Onions and tomatoes lose 75 to 80 percent of their initial quercetin content after boiling for fifteen minutes; 65 percent after cooking in a microwave oven, and 30 percent after frying. Choose raw or lightly steamed vegetables to minimize vital nutrients lost in cooking.

> It is important to buy local produce when possible so that the time between harvest and purchase is kept to a minimum.

Studies have repeatedly shown the risk of chronic disease goes down as the consumption of a diet rich in polyphenols goes up. Consumption of antioxidants has been linked to reduced levels of oxidative cell damage. Evidence is mounting that polyphenols act as antioxidants to protect our cells and, therefore, can prevent degenerative diseases associated with oxidative stress.

Top Food Sources of Polyphenols

In a study recently published in the *Journal of Nutrition* (Zamora-Ros et al., 2013), researchers have determined that including more than 650 milligrams of polyphenols a day in your diet increases longevity by 30 percent. As you can see from the chart, many foods listed contain multiple types and varying amounts of polyphenols. For example, 100 grams of blueberries could give you over 750 milligrams of polyphenols per serving. While it would be tedious to calculate your polyphenol intake daily, I have included this chart as a reference tool for you to determine which foods to include in order to receive the highest polyphenol benefit.

Polyphenols in Food

Type of Polyphenol	Serving Size (100 g)	Amount of Polyphenol (mg/serving)
Hydroxybenzoic acids	Blackberry	8–27
	Raspberry	6–10
	Strawberry	2–9
Hydroxycinnamic acids	Blueberry	200–220
	Kiwi	60–100
	Cherry	18–115
	Plum	14–115
	Apple	5–60
	Pear	1.5–60
	Potato	10–19
	Corn flour	30.5
	Flour: wheat, rice, oat	6.5–9
	Coffee (100mL)	35–175
Anthocyanins	Blackberry	100–400
	Blueberry	25–500
	Black grape	30–750
	Cherry	35–450
	Rhubarb	200
	Strawberry	15–75
	Red wine (100mL)	20–35
	Plum	2–25
	Red cabbage	25
Flavonols	Yellow onion	35–120
	Curly kale	30–60
	Leek	3–22.5
	Cherry tomato	1.5–20
	Broccoli	4–10
	Blueberry	3–16
	Apricot	2.5–5
	Apple	2–4
	Beans, green or white	1–5
	Black grape	1.5–4
	Tomato	0.2–1.5
	Black tea infusion (100mL)	3–4.5
	Green tea infusion (100mL)	2–3.5
	Red wine (100mL)	0.2–3

continued on next page

Type of Polyphenol	Serving Size (100 g)	Amount of Polyphenol (mg/serving)
Flavones	Parsley	24–184
	Celery	2–14
	Capsicum pepper	0.5–1
Flavanones	Orange juice (100mL)	20–70
	Grapefruit juice (100mL)	10–65
	Lemon juice (100mL)	5–30
Isoflavones	Soy flour	78–175.5
	Soybeans, boiled	20–90
	Miso	25–90
	Tofu	8–70
	Soy milk (100mL)	3–17.5
Monomeric flavanols	Chocolate	46–60
	Beans	35–55
	Apricot	10–25
	Cherry	5–22
	Grape	3–17.5
	Peach	5–14
	Blackberry	13
	Apple	2–12
	Green tea (100mL)	10–80
	Black tea (100mL)	6–50
	Red wine (100mL)	8–30

Adapted from: Manach, C., Scalbert, A., Morand, C., Remesy, C., and Jimenez, L. "Polyphenols: Food Sources and Bioavailability." *American Journal of Clinical Nutrition* 79, 5 (2004): 727-47.

Additional Anti-Inflammatory Micronutrients

In addition to polyphenols, there are many other micronutrients in foods that are known to be extremely beneficial in keeping us free from chronic disease.

A great resource for these and other powerful AI sources is discussed on the *CanSurvive Cuisine* website at www.cansurvivecuisine.com.

- Terpenes (such as perillyl alcohol, limonene, and carnosol) may protect cells from becoming cancerous; slow cancer cell growth; strengthen immune function; limit production of cancer-related hormones; fight viruses; and work as antioxidants. Some examples of foods containing terpenes are cherries, citrus fruit peel, and rosemary.

- Isothiocyanates may induce detoxification of carcinogens, block tumor growth, and work as antioxidants. Some examples of foods containing isothiocyanates are cruciferous vegetables such as broccoli, cabbage, collard greens, kale, cauliflower, and Brussels sprouts.

- Isoflavones may inhibit tumor growth, limit production of cancer-related hormones, and generally work as antioxidants. Some examples of foods containing isoflavones are soybeans and soy products (tofu, soy milk, and edamame).

- Inositol may retard cell growth and work as an antioxidant. Some examples of foods containing inositol are bran from corn, oats, rice, rye, and wheat; nuts; and soybeans and soy products.

- Indoles and glucosinolates may induce detoxification of carcinogens, block carcinogens, and prevent tumor growth. Food sources include cruciferous vegetables.

There have been many fascinating studies on individual foods and micronutrients to determine their contribution to helping avoid inflammation. I could fill the next thousand pages giving you sample studies; however, this book is about sifting through the science to make AI user-friendly, so I will summarize a few super-exciting studies and break the science into usable pieces to make anti-inflammatory practical for you to use in your everyday life.

●　●　●

One powerful study is the review article done by Galland (2010). In the review, he states that chronic inflammation is involved in both development and progression of degenerative disease. He notes that a diet high in healthy fats, fruits, vegetables, legumes, and grains has a measurable anti-inflammatory effect on our body. Eating to lessen chronic inflammation gives us a powerful tool to help prevent some of the most devastating chronic diseases. A more thorough review of this study can be found in the Appendix.

●　●　●

Other exciting research is in a small study done recently on the impact of implementing an anti-inflammatory diet on cognitive decline (Bredesen et al., 2014). The intervention in this study is a personalized program based on the disease process involved in Alzheimer's patients. Multiple lifestyle interventions provided dramatic "metabolic enhancement for neurodegeneration (MEND)." Ten people involved in the study included patients with Alzheimer's disease (AD) and those with other cognitive impairments. Nine of the ten achieved improvement in cognition in 3–6 months; the only exception was a patient with late-stage Alzheimer's. These improvements continued for two and one-half years from the initial treatment. Based on these findings, a larger study is warranted. Further, the results may mean that early-stage cognitive decline may be stopped or even reversed with dietary intervention.

•   •   •

A recent study published in *Diabetes Care* was designed to determine if a pistachio-rich diet reduces the prediabetes stage (Hernandez-Alonso et al., 2014). Fasting glucose, insulin, and insulin resistance decreased significantly after the pistachio diet. Data suggest that pistachios are anti-inflammatory and lower glucose and insulin. Thus, this dietary intervention can reverse certain metabolic harmful effects of prediabetes.

•   •   •

For those of you who love the science and want more, I've created a list of several of my favorite studies, listed by their chronic disease state, along with a brief description and a link where you can see the study in its entirety. These favorites can be found in the Appendix.

Scientific evidence is growing to strongly suggest a link between diet, inflammation, and disease. From studies such as these, our understanding of the role between diet, lifestyle, and chronic disease will continue to develop. The good news is that there are things you can do NOW to take charge of your health and improve your quality of life.

Recipes

I'm a business owner, public speaker, and dietitian. I'm also a foodie, a mother, a wife, a grandmother, and a dinner party guru! I want the food I serve—and enjoy—to taste delicious AND promote good health. These recipes will help you make meals for your family and friends that will do both! **—Jan Tilley**

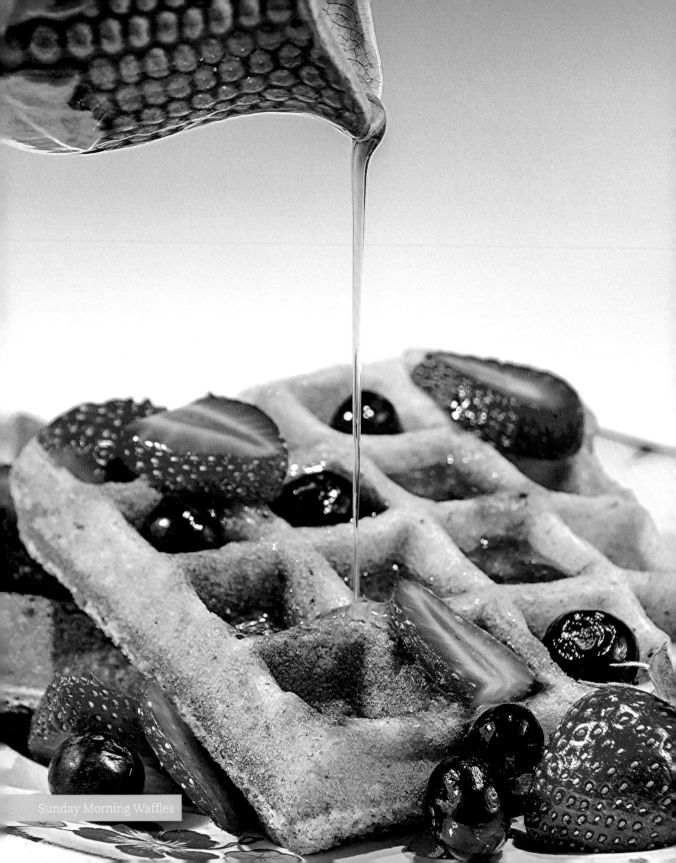

Sunday Morning Waffles

Sunday Morning Waffles

Makes 8 waffles.

Ingredients:

1 cup whole wheat flour

1 tablespoon ground flaxseed

1 tablespoon sugar

1 heaping teaspoon baking powder

½ teaspoon baking soda

¼ teaspoon salt

1 ½ cups low-fat buttermilk, divided

1 egg

¼ cup canola oil

Directions:

1. In large bowl, combine flour, flaxseed, sugar, baking powder, baking soda, and salt.

2. Add 1 cup buttermilk and egg, and whisk until smooth. Let stand 15 minutes.

3. Add remaining ½ cup buttermilk and oil; whisk until smooth.

4. Pour batter into preheated waffle iron sprayed with cooking spray. Serve immediately.

Nutrition Information: 160 calories, 9 grams fat, 30 mg cholesterol, 320 mg sodium, 16 grams carbohydrate, 2 grams fiber, 4 grams protein

Exchanges: 1 Carbohydrate, 0.5 Protein, 2 Fat

Did you know whole grains act as a prebiotic to fuel healthy bacteria in your gut?

Chilled Banana-Berry Oatmeal

Makes 1 serving.

½ banana

¼ cup dry rolled oats

⅓ cup low-fat vanilla Greek yogurt

¼ cup water

1 tablespoon walnuts, chopped

¼ cup blueberries

1. In a medium bowl, mash banana and stir in oats, Greek yogurt, and water. Cover and refrigerate overnight.

2. In the morning, stir and serve with chopped walnuts and blueberries.

Nutrition Information: 250 calories, 8g fat, 5mg cholesterol, 55mg sodium, 38g carbohydrate, 5g fiber, 9g protein

Exchanges: 2.5 Carbohydrates, 1 Protein, 1.5 Fat

Try adding 1 teaspoon of dark unsweetened cocoa powder to boost AI benefit in this easy breakfast treat!

Farmer's Breakfast

Makes 8 servings.

8 eggs, lightly beaten

¼ cup 1% milk

2 tablespoons fresh parsley, snipped

½ teaspoon each salt and fresh ground black pepper

6 small red new potatoes, quartered

2 tablespoons canola oil

1 cup fresh mushrooms, quartered

1 cup turkey or soy sausage crumbles

1 small green pepper, chopped

½ cup onion, chopped

1 cup low-fat cheddar cheese shreds

1. In medium bowl, combine eggs, milk, parsley, salt, and black pepper; set aside.

2. In large nonstick skillet, cook potatoes in oil over medium-high heat for 10-12 minutes or until browned, turning occasionally.

3. Add mushrooms, sausage crumbles, green pepper, and onion. Cook and stir for 5-8 minutes or until vegetables are just tender. Reduce heat to low and add egg mixture to skillet.

4. Cook, stirring occasionally, until eggs begin to set. Sprinkle with cheese and continue cooking until eggs are desired consistency.

Nutrition Information: 190 calories, 10g fat, 220mg cholesterol, 440mg sodium, 9g carbohydrate, 1g fiber, 14g protein

Exchanges: 0.5 Carbohydrates, 2 Protein, 2 Fat

Everyday Egg Soufflés

Makes 12 servings.

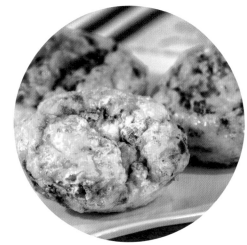

6 eggs

6 egg whites (discard yolks or use in another recipe)

2 tablespoons Parmesan cheese

¼ teaspoon each salt and fresh ground black pepper

½ cup fresh spinach, chopped

½ cup thinly sliced mushrooms

½ cup low-fat cheese shreds

Optional: diced jalapeño, diced green onion, diced tomato

Everyday Egg Soufflés

1. Preheat oven to 350 degrees. Prepare 12 large muffin tins by spraying with cooking spray.

2. In large bowl, whisk together eggs, egg whites, Parmesan cheese, salt, and pepper.

3. Fill tins with half of the egg mixture. Top with equal portions of spinach, mushrooms, and cheese shreds. Add jalapeños, green onions, and tomato, if desired. Top evenly with remaining egg mixture.

4. Bake for 22-25 minutes. Remove from muffin tins and serve or cool on wire rack and wrap in plastic wrap. Store in refrigerator for up to one week. Remove one or two for breakfast, heat in microwave for about 30 seconds, and breakfast is ready!

Nutrition Information: 60 calories, 3g fat, 110mg cholesterol, 180mg sodium, 1g carbohydrate, 0g fiber, 7g protein

Exchanges: 0 Carbohydrate, 1 Protein, 0.5 Fat

Jan's Famous Zucchini Muffins

Makes 28 muffins.

3 eggs

¾ cup canola oil

1 tablespoon vanilla

3 cups shredded zucchini

1 cup brown sugar

2 cups whole wheat flour

2 teaspoons cinnamon

1 ½ teaspoons baking soda

1 teaspoon salt

¼ teaspoon baking powder

1. Preheat oven to 400 degrees. Spray muffin tin with cooking spray.

2. In large bowl, combine eggs, oil, vanilla, and zucchini. In a separate medium bowl, combine dry ingredients; add to zucchini mixture and stir until just moistened.

3. Fill muffin tins ⅔ full and bake at 400 degrees for 18 minutes.

Nutrition Information: 120 calories, 7g fat, 25mg cholesterol, 170mg sodium, 14g carbohydrate, 1g fiber, 2g protein

Exchanges: 1 Carbohydrates, 0.5 Protein, 1 Fat

Cinnamon is best known for its warm flavor and cozy, sultry aroma. However, cinnamon is also a potent antioxidant and anti-inflammatory agent. While cinnamon pairs well with sweet foods and can be enjoyed sprinkled over oatmeal, in coffee, or on fresh fruit, it can also jazz up your favorite savory meals. Try it on roasted root vegetables!

Strawberry Banana Smoothie

Makes 1 serving.

½ cup plain 0% fat Greek yogurt

¼ cup unsweetened light almond milk (or low-fat milk)

½ banana

¼ cup mixed frozen berries

1 teaspoon ground flaxseed

1. Combine all ingredients in blender (or other smoothie maker).
2. Whirl together until blended.

Nutrition Information: 150 calories, 2g fat, 0mg cholesterol, 90mg sodium, 23g carbohydrate, 4g fiber, 12g protein

Exchanges: 1.5 Carbohydrate, 1.5 Protein, .5 Fat

Go bananas! This creamy fruit is a heart-healthy source of soluble fiber gift-wrapped by nature for an easy, portable, anti-inflammatory snack.

Mega-Nutrient Smoothie

Makes 1 serving.

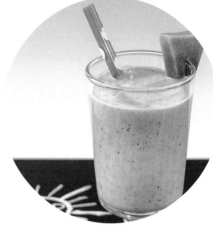

- ½ cup unsweetened light almond milk (or 1% milk)
- ¾ cup kale
- ½ cup plain 0% fat Greek yogurt
- ½ banana, frozen
- ¼ cup papaya
- ¼ cup strawberries
- 1 tablespoon almond butter

1. Combine all ingredients in blender or smoothie maker.
2. Whirl together until well blended.

Mega-Nutrient Smoothie

Nutrition Information: 260 calories, 11g fat, 0mg cholesterol, 180mg sodium, 28g carbohydrate, 5g fiber, 15g protein

Exchanges: 2 Carbohydrate, 2 Protein, 2 Fat

I challenged my team to create a smoothie using food, not supplements, to supercharge your day. Enjoy this treat as your good-morning "Health in a Glass!"

Rolled Omelet

Makes 12 servings.

4 ounces reduced-fat cream cheese

¾ cup 1% milk

2 tablespoons all-purpose flour

¼ teaspoon each salt and fresh ground black pepper

2 tablespoons Dijon mustard

12 eggs

2 cups reduced-fat Cheddar cheese shreds, divided

1 cup finely diced low-sodium uncured ham

¼ cup thinly sliced green onions

Optional: salsa

1. Preheat oven to 375 degrees. Line greased 15x10-inch baking pan with parchment paper; spray paper with cooking spray and set aside.

2. In large bowl, beat cream cheese and milk until smooth. Add flour, salt, pepper, and mustard; mix until smooth. Add eggs and blend well. Pour into prepared pan and place carefully into oven.

3. Bake for 25 to 30 minutes or until eggs are puffed and set. Remove from oven and sprinkle with 1 cup of cheese, ham, and onions. Top with remaining cheese, reserving ¼ cup to sprinkle on top of roll.

4. Roll omelet from short side, peeling parchment paper away while rolling. Sprinkle top of roll with remaining cheese; bake an additional 3 to 5 minutes or until cheese is melted. Serve with salsa, if desired.

Nutrition Information: 180 calories, 11g fat, 235mg cholesterol, 460mg sodium, 3g carbohydrate, 0g fiber, 16g protein

Exchanges: 0 carbohydrate, 2.5 protein, 2 fat

For an extra AI benefit, finely chop an assortment of your favorite veggies and add with the cheese in place of ham.

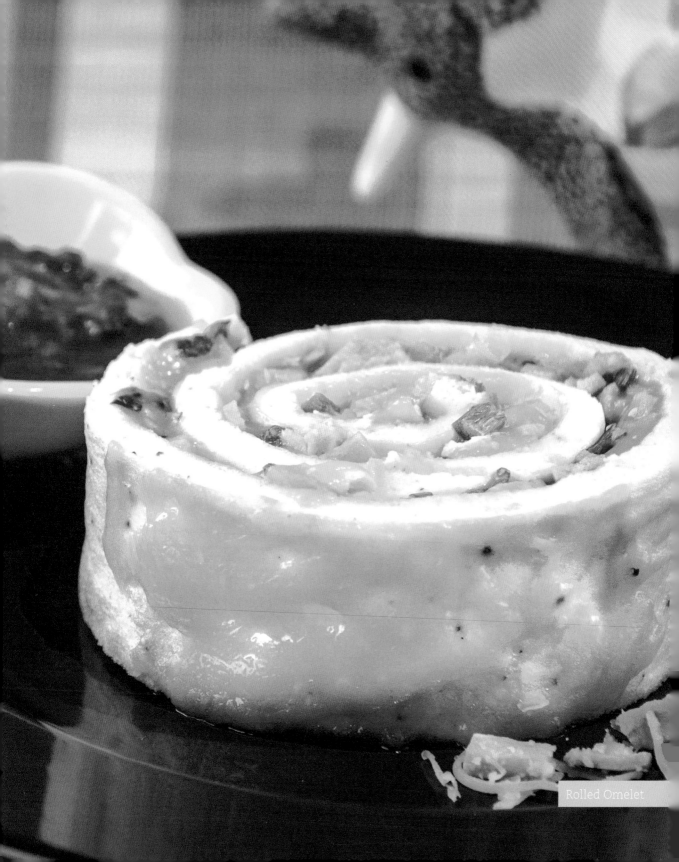

Rolled Omelet

Vegetable Frittata

Makes 6 servings.

1 tablespoon olive oil

½ cup finely diced red new potatoes

½ cup sliced mushrooms

½ cup diced zucchini

2 green onions, thinly sliced

2 tablespoons diced jalapeños

1 cup fresh baby spinach

6 eggs, slightly beaten

¼ cup 1% milk

1 cup reduced-fat Cheddar cheese shreds

2 tablespoons Parmesan cheese shreds

½ teaspoon each salt and fresh ground black pepper

Optional Toppings: halved cherry tomatoes, diced avocado, salsa

1. In large, oven-proof skillet, heat olive oil over medium heat. Sauté potatoes, mushrooms, and zucchini for 5 minutes, stirring often. Add green onions, jalapeños, and spinach; cook for 1 minute. Remove skillet from stove top and set aside.

2. In medium bowl, whisk together eggs, milk, cheeses, salt, and pepper. Pour carefully over vegetable mixture in skillet. Use light strokes with fork to help incorporate egg into vegetable mixture.

3. Bake at 350 degrees for 20 minutes or until frittata is set in the center.

Nutrition information: 180 calories, 11g fat, 225mg cholesterol, 450mg sodium, 5g carbohydrate, 1g fiber, 13g protein

Exchanges: 0.5 Carbohydrate, 2 Protein, 2 Fat

Tomato, Spinach & Feta Strata

Makes 6 servings.

3 cups cubed sourdough bread

1 pound fresh asparagus, trimmed and cut into 1-inch pieces

1 cup chopped onion

2 cups fresh baby spinach

6 eggs

1 cup 1% milk

⅛ teaspoon each salt and fresh ground black pepper

2 plum tomatoes, thinly sliced

½ cup reduced-fat feta cheese

¼ cup snipped fresh basil

1. Coat a 2-quart rectangular baking dish with cooking spray. Arrange half of the bread cubes in the prepared baking dish.

2. In a medium saucepan, bring 4 cups of water to boil. Add asparagus and onion and cook for 2 to 3 minutes or just until tender; stir in spinach and immediately drain well. Spoon half of the asparagus mixture over bread in baking dish. Top with the remaining bread cubes and the remaining asparagus mixture. Set aside.

3. In a large bowl, whisk together eggs, milk, salt, and pepper. Pour evenly over mixture in baking dish. With the back of a large spoon, lightly press down layers. Arrange tomato slices on top. Sprinkle with feta cheese and basil. Cover with foil; refrigerate overnight or up to 24 hours.

4. Preheat oven to 325 degrees. Bake, covered, for 30 minutes. Uncover; bake about 30 minutes more or until center is set. Let stand on a wire rack for 10 minutes before serving.

Nutrition Information: 210 calories, 9g fat, 235 mg cholesterol, 410 mg sodium, 21g carbohydrate, 3g fiber, 14g protein

Exchanges: 1.5 Carbohydrate, 2 Protein, 2 Fat

Fresh basil is a natural anti-inflammatory. It has been shown to inhibit the same enzyme targeted by the anti-inflammatory drug, ibuprofen.

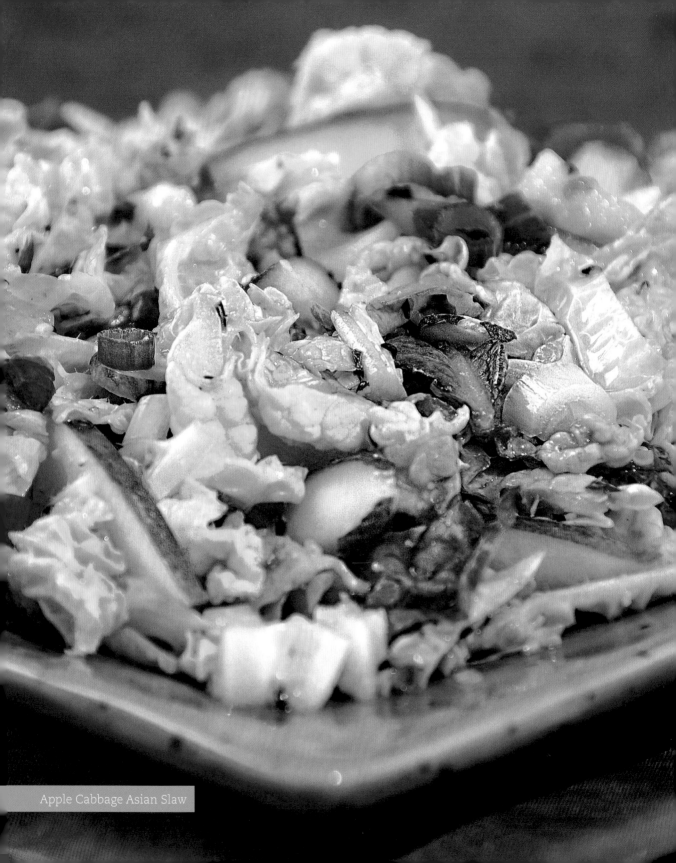

Apple Cabbage Asian Slaw

Apple Cabbage Asian Slaw

Makes 8 servings.

Ingredients:

Salad:

1 head (approximately 8 cups)
    Napa cabbage, shredded

1 Red Delicious apple, julienned

1 green onion, thinly sliced

2 tablespoons cilantro, chopped

¼ cup almonds, sliced

2 tablespoons hemp seeds, raw

½ teaspoon salt

¼ teaspoon fresh ground black pepper

Dressing:

⅓ cup extra-virgin olive oil

¼ cup rice vinegar

2 tablespoons tamari

1 tablespoon fresh ginger, minced

2 cloves garlic, minced

1 teaspoon honey

Directions:

1. Combine all salad ingredients into a large bowl, toss together, and set aside.
2. In small bowl, whisk together all of the dressing ingredients until well blended.
3. Pour dressing over salad mixture, toss, and serve.

Nutrition Information: 160 calories, 12g fat, 0mg cholesterol, 410mg sodium, 11g carbohydrate, 2g fiber, 3g protein

Exchanges: 0.5 Carbohydrate, 0.5 Protein, 2.5 Fat

Hemp seeds are an excellent source of protein, insoluble fiber, and omega-3 fatty acids. Blend in smoothies, mix in yogurt, or add to baked goods and hot cereal. Hemp seeds are readily available at most supermarkets.

Confetti Broccoli Salad

Makes 8 servings.

⅓ cup dried cranberries

⅓ cup slivered almonds, toasted

2 slices center-cut bacon, fried crisp
  and crumbled

¼ cup green onions, chopped

4 cups broccoli florets

½ cup red bell pepper, chopped

½ cup grated carrots

1 ½ tablespoons sugar

¼ cup red wine vinegar

3 tablespoons canola oil

1. In large bowl, combine dried cranberries, almonds, bacon crumbles, green onions, broccoli, red bell pepper, and carrots; set aside.

2. In small bowl, whisk together sugar, vinegar, and canola oil.

3. Pour dressing over broccoli mixture and stir. Place in refrigerator overnight to allow flavors to marinate.

Nutrition Information: 120 calories, 8g fat, 0mg cholesterol, 50mg sodium,
  10g carbohydrate, 2g fiber, 3g protein

Exchanges: 1 Carbohydrate, 0.5 Protein, 1.5 Fat

Almonds are rich in monounsaturated fatty acids, dietary fiber, biotin, and vitamin E! This heart-healthy snack can be enjoyed on its own, in hot cereal, yogurt, baked goods, or sprinkled on a salad.

Corn & Black Bean Salad

Makes 8 servings.

2 cups fresh roasted corn kernels
(approximately 4 ears) or 1 (8 oz.)
can summer crisp corn, drained

1 red bell pepper, diced

¼ cup thinly sliced green onions

¼ cup fresh cilantro, chopped

1 (15 oz.) can black beans, rinsed
and drained

3 tablespoons lime juice

2 teaspoons canola oil

½ teaspoon each garlic powder, ground
cumin, chili powder, and fresh
ground black pepper

Dash of salt

1 small avocado, diced

1. Combine corn, bell pepper, green onions, cilantro, and beans in a medium bowl.

2. Combine lime juice, oil, and seasonings in a small bowl. Drizzle over corn mixture; toss
well. Gently stir in avocado. Cover and chill 30 minutes.

Nutrition Information: 140 calories, 5g fat, 0mg cholesterol, 200mg sodium,
22g carbohydrate, 5g fiber, 5g protein

Exchanges: 1.5 Carbohydrate, 1 Protein, 1 Fat

Looking for the perfect AI dish—this may just be it!

Chipotle Chicken Taco Salad

Makes 6 servings.

Dressing:

- ¼ cup chopped fresh cilantro
- ½ cup fat-free plain Greek yogurt
- 1 tablespoon minced chipotle chile, canned in adobo
- 1 teaspoon each ground cumin and chili powder
- 2 tablespoons fresh lime juice
- ¼ teaspoon each salt and freshly ground black pepper

Salad:

- 4 cups shredded romaine lettuce
- 3 cups cooked chicken breasts, cut into cubes
- 1 cup cherry tomatoes, halved
- 1 small avocado, peeled and cut into cubes
- ¼ cup vertically sliced red onion
- 1 (15 oz.) can black beans, rinsed and drained
- 1 (8 ¾ oz.) can summer crisp corn, rinsed and drained
- ½ cup chopped mango

1. To prepare dressing: In small bowl, combine all dressing ingredients. Whisk and place in refrigerator.

2. To prepare salad: In large serving bowl, combine lettuce and remaining ingredients. Drizzle dressing over salad; toss gently to coat. Serve immediately.

Nutrition Information: 240 calories, 6g fat, 30mg cholesterol, 370mg sodium, 27g carbohydrate, 10g fiber, 20g protein

Exchanges: 2 Carbohydrate, 3 Protein, 1 Fat

Black beans are a healthy choice high in fiber and protein. These AI powerhouses are an inexpensive and delicious addition to your favorite salad, salsa, and soup recipes.

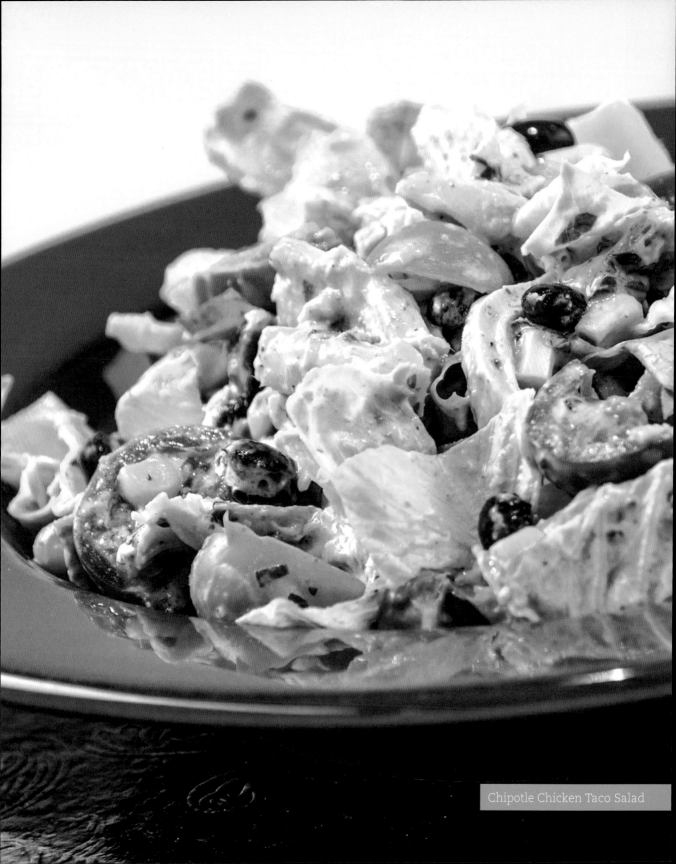

Chipotle Chicken Taco Salad

Cranberry Pecan Chicken Salad

Makes 6 servings.

- ⅓ cup toasted pecans, chopped
- 3 cups chopped cooked boneless, skinless chicken breast
- ⅓ cup dried cranberries
- 2 celery ribs, finely chopped
- ½ cup light mayonnaise
- 1 tablespoon Cavender's All-Purpose Greek Seasoning
- 2 tablespoons fresh lemon juice
- Optional: 6 cups of spinach

1. Stir together pecans, chicken, dried cranberries, celery, mayonnaise, Greek seasoning, and lemon juice.
2. Place chicken salad on bed of spinach, if desired, and serve. May cover and refrigerate to serve later.

Nutrition Information: 240 calories, 12g fat, 65mg cholesterol, 310mg sodium, 9g carbohydrate, 1g fiber, 23g protein

Exchanges: 0.5 Carbohydrate, 3 Protein, 2 Fat

Pecans are a great source of omega-6 fatty acids, dietary fiber, and protein. Eating a handful of pecans every day has been shown to lower cholesterol levels as much as some medications.

Salads

Layered Chicken Salad

Makes 6 servings.

Salad:

4 cups romaine lettuce, chopped

1 ½ cups broccoli florets

1 ½ cups cauliflower florets

¼ cup green onion, chopped

1 cup green seedless grapes

2 cups cooked chicken breast, chopped

½ cup reduced-fat feta cheese crumbles

¼ cup sliced almonds, toasted

Dressing:

½ cup light mayonnaise

3 tablespoons low-sugar orange marmalade

½ cup plain 0% fat Greek yogurt

1. In large glass bowl, layer salad ingredients in order listed, reserving feta crumbles and almonds.

2. To prepare dressing, in small bowl whisk together mayonnaise, marmalade, and yogurt.

3. Spread dressing over chicken, top with feta crumbles and sliced almonds.
   May be prepared up to a day before. Toss gently just before serving.

Nutrition Information: 160 calories, 5g fat, 45mg cholesterol, 210mg sodium, 10g carbohydrate, 3g fiber, 19g protein

Exchanges: 1 carbohydrate, 3 protein, 1 fat

Kale & Quinoa Salad

Makes 8 servings.

1 (8.5 oz) package microwavable quinoa & brown rice blend

6 cups baby kale

3 tablespoons olive oil

3 tablespoons fresh lemon juice

1 tablespoon Dijon mustard

½ teaspoon each fresh ground black pepper and salt

¼ cup coarsely chopped pecans

¼ cup dried cranberries

¼ cup reduced-fat feta cheese

1. Microwave quinoa and rice blend according to package directions and allow to cool.

2. Roughly chop kale; place in large salad bowl.

3. In a small bowl, whisk together olive oil, lemon juice, Dijon mustard, pepper, and salt. Drizzle dressing over kale.

4. Add cooled quinoa blend, pecans, dried cranberries, and feta to the dressed kale and toss well.

Nutrition Information: 150 calories, 9g fat, 0mg cholesterol, 340mg sodium, 15g carbohydrate, 2g fiber, 3g protein

Exchanges: 1 Carbohydrate, 0.5 Protein, 2 Fat

Need a massage? Kale is an incredibly nutrient-rich, high-fiber, green leafy vegetable that has a bad reputation of being tough and bitter. It doesn't have to be! After chopping, firmly massage the kale leaves until darker green and silky in texture. While it may seem odd to massage your food, a few minutes of special attention can make all the difference!

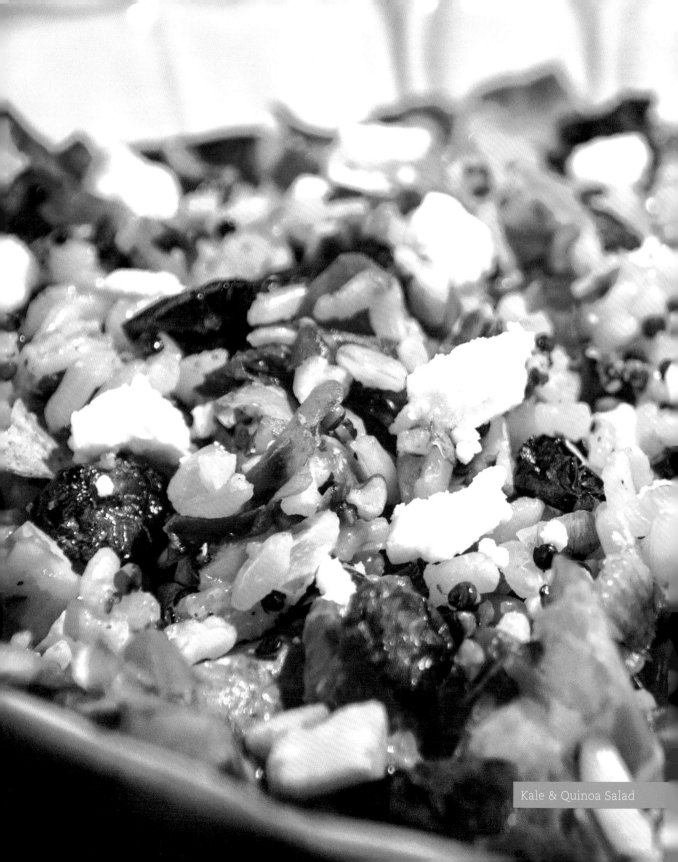

Kale & Quinoa Salad

Crunchy Apple Chicken Salad

Makes 4 servings.

Salad:

4 (approximately 4 oz. each) cooked boneless skinless chicken breast halves

1 cup diced red apple

1 cup chopped celery

⅓ cup sliced almonds, toasted

Dressing:

½ cup plain 0% fat Greek yogurt

2 tablespoons light mayonnaise

1 tablespoon honey

1 tablespoon fresh lemon juice

¼ teaspoon each salt and white pepper

4 large lettuce leaves

1. Cut chicken into bite-size pieces. Combine chicken, apple, celery, and almonds in a large bowl; set aside.

2. To prepare dressing: whisk together yogurt, mayonnaise, honey, lemon juice, salt, and white pepper in a small bowl. Add dressing to chicken mixture and toss gently to coat.

3. Store in refrigerator until ready to serve. Place lettuce leaves on four individual serving plates, top with chicken salad, and serve.

Nutrition Information: 260 calories, 10g fat, 65mg cholesterol, 280mg sodium, 13g carbohydrate, 2g fiber, 28g protein

Exchanges: 1 Carbohydrate, 4 Protein, 2 Fat

Greek Pasta Salad

Makes 8 servings.

Marinade:

1 tablespoon olive oil

1 tablespoon fresh lemon juice

1 teaspoon ground fennel seeds

1 teaspoon dried oregano

¼ teaspoon salt

Dash of fresh ground black pepper

Salad:

1 (15 oz.) can chickpeas, rinsed and drained

1 tablespoon olive oil

2 tablespoons minced or pressed garlic

½ cup diced celery

1 red bell pepper, seeded and diced

1 ½ cups diced tomatoes

½ cup finely chopped green onion

8 ounces whole grain penne pasta

12 pitted chopped Kalamata olives, chopped

¼ cup chopped fresh parsley

2 tablespoons fresh lemon juice

1 cup crumbled reduced-fat feta cheese

1. Whisk together all of the marinade ingredients in a medium bowl. Add the chickpeas and set aside.

2. Heat oil in a large skillet over medium heat; add garlic and gently sauté until just golden, a minute or two. Add the celery, bell peppers, and tomatoes and continue to cook, stirring occasionally, for about 10 minutes. Stir in the green onion and marinated chickpeas; cook for about 3 minutes.

3. While vegetables are cooking, bring water to a boil in large pot. Add pasta to boiling water and cook until al dente; drain well. Transfer the pasta to a large serving bowl and add the sautéed vegetables, olives, parsley, and lemon juice. Toss well.

4. Top with feta cheese and serve warm or chilled.

Nutrition Information: 240 calories, 9g fat, 15mg cholesterol, 430mg sodium, 34g carbohydrates, 6g fiber, 11g protein

Exchanges: 2 Carbohydrates, 1.5 Protein, 2 Fat

Fennel seeds are potent sources of the anti-inflammatory and antioxidant compound called anethole. This unique spice has a flavor very similar to that of licorice and anise, and is a delicious addition to salads, yogurt, or seafood.

Vietnamese Spring Roll Salad

Makes 4 servings.

Salad:

- 4 ounces vermicelli rice noodles, cooked as directed on package
- 2 cups skinless, cold rotisserie chicken breast, shredded
- 2 cups Boston lettuce, torn
- 1 cup matchstick carrots
- 1 cup fresh bean sprouts
- 1 red bell pepper, thinly sliced
- 2 green onions, sliced
- 1 cup fresh papaya, cubed
- ¼ cup each basil, cilantro, and mint, roughly chopped
- ¼ cup unsalted, dry roasted peanuts, coarsely chopped
- 1 jalapeño, seeded and sliced

Peanut Dressing:

- ½ teaspoon canola oil
- 1 clove garlic, minced
- 2 tablespoons peanut butter
- 1 tablespoons hoisin sauce
- ¼ cup water
- ½ teaspoon fish sauce or low-sodium soy sauce
- ½ teaspoon brown sugar
- 1 fresh lime, juiced
- 1 teaspoon sriracha chili sauce

1. Assemble salad ingredients in large bowl. Place in refrigerator while preparing the dressing.
2. To prepare dressing, heat oil in pan over medium heat, add garlic and sauté until fragrant. Add remaining ingredients and simmer over low heat until mixture thickens, about 2 minutes. Let cool; then toss with salad and serve.

Nutrition Information: 370 calories, 12g fat, 50mg cholesterol, 420mg sodium, 45g carbohydrate, 6g fiber, 26g protein

Exchanges: 3 Carbohydrate, 4 Protein, 2.5 Fat

Basil is a highly fragrant herb known for its anti-microbial and anti-inflammatory characteristics. In addition to being the perfect companion to Italian dishes, basil can be added to your favorite Asian dishes for extra flair and nutritional value.

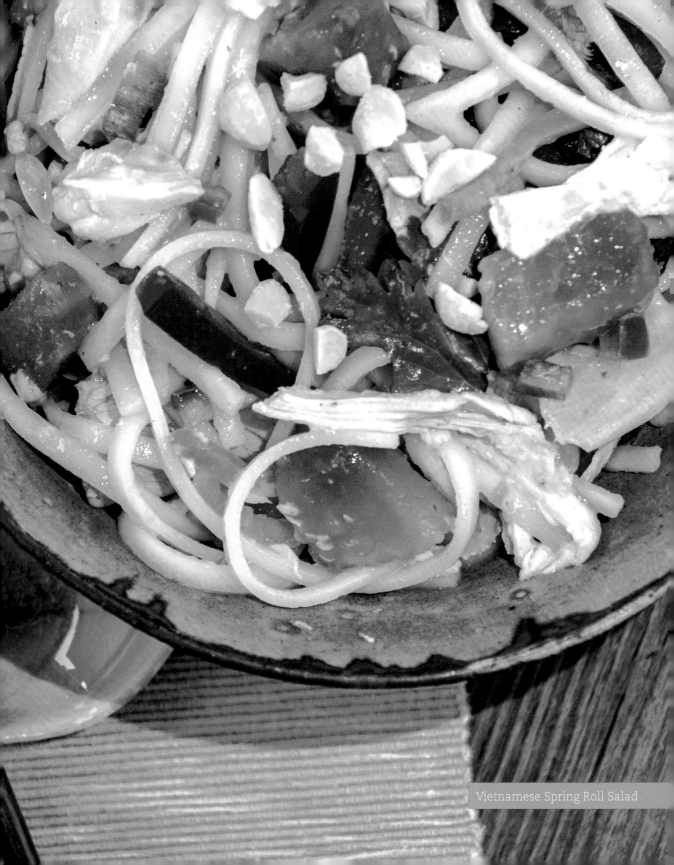

Vietnamese Spring Roll Salad

Tuna Salad on Fresh Baby Spinach

Makes 6 servings.

2 (5 oz. cans) albacore tuna (packed in water), drained

2 hard-boiled eggs, chopped

½ cup finely chopped celery

½ cup finely chopped apple

¼ cup spicy sweet pickles, chopped + 1 tablespoon pickle juice

¼ cup toasted pecans, chopped

½ cup light mayonnaise

1 tablespoon Dijon mustard

¼ teaspoon each salt and fresh ground black pepper

8 cups baby spinach

Optional: cherry tomatoes, light balsamic vinaigrette

1. In large bowl, combine tuna, egg, celery, apple, sweet pickles, and pecans.

2. Add light mayonnaise, Dijon mustard, salt, and pepper. Stir together and refrigerate until ready to use.

3. To prepare salad, place 2 cups of baby spinach on 4 individual serving plates. Place a 1-cup mound of tuna salad on top of spinach. Serve with cherry tomatoes and a 1-tablespoon drizzle of light balsamic vinaigrette, if desired.

Nutrition Information: 210 calories, 13g fat, 100mg cholesterol, 430mg sodium, 9g carbohydrate, 3g fiber, 15g protein

Exchanges: 0.5 Carbohydrate, 2 Protein, 2.5 Fat

Zesty Tex-Mex Watermelon Salad

Makes 6 servings.

Salad:

- 5 cups cubed seedless watermelon, cut into 1-inch pieces
- 1 cup cubed cucumber, peeled and seeded
- ¼ cup thinly-sliced red onion
- 1 jalapeño pepper, seeded and finely chopped
- ¼ cup each fresh cilantro and mint, chopped
- ½ cup crumbled reduced-fat feta cheese

Vinaigrette:

- 2 tablespoons fresh lime juice
- Zest of 1 lime
- 1 tablespoons extra-virgin olive oil
- 1 tablespoon honey
- ¼ teaspoon each sea salt and fresh cracked pepper

1. In a large bowl, place watermelon, cucumber, red onion, jalapeño, cilantro, and mint. Reserve feta to add before serving.

2. To prepare vinaigrette, whisk together lime juice, lime zest, olive oil, and honey in a small bowl. Season with salt and pepper and set aside.

3. Just before serving, drain any excess liquid from watermelon mixture. Add vinaigrette and feta cheese to the salad and toss lightly to coat.

Nutrition Information: 110 calories, 4g fat, 5mg cholesterol, 270mg sodium, 16g carbohydrate, 2g fiber, 4g protein

Exchanges: 1 Carbohydrate, 0.5 Protein, 1 Fat

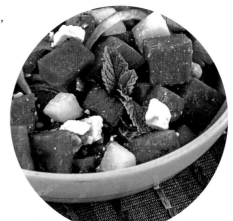

Zesty Tex-Mex Watermelon Salad

Watermelon contains phenolic compounds, making this fruit deliciously anti-inflammatory and anti-oxidant rich. To enjoy the maximum health benefits from this juicy summer treat, select a ripe melon that is heavy for its size, has smooth skin, and has a yellow-cream colored underbelly.

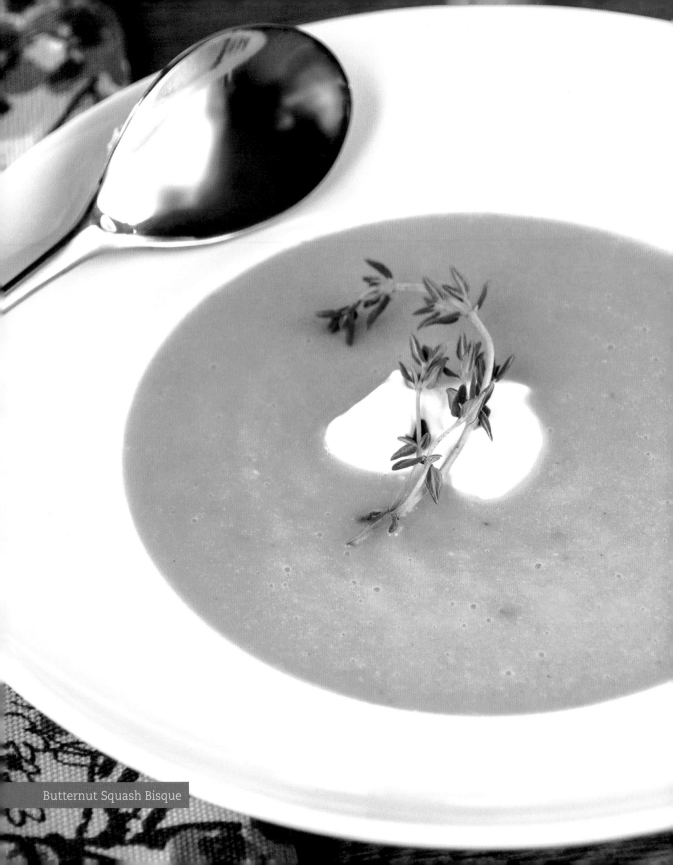

Butternut Squash Bisque

Butternut Squash Bisque

Makes 8 servings.

Ingredients:

2 butternut squash, halved & seeded

1 large unpeeled onion

1 small garlic bulb

2 tablespoons olive oil

2 tablespoons minced fresh thyme or 2 teaspoons dried thyme

3 cups organic chicken broth

¼ cup heavy whipping cream

½ teaspoon salt

¼ teaspoon each seasoned salt & fresh ground white pepper

Optional: sprigs fresh thyme

Directions:

1. Place squash cut side up on 15 × 10 × 1-inch baking pan. Cut ¼ inch off tops of onion and garlic bulbs (the end that comes to a closed point) and place cut side up in baking pans. Brush with oil; sprinkle with thyme. Cover pan tightly with aluminum foil and bake at 350 degrees for 1-½ to 2 hours or until vegetables are very tender. Uncover and let stand until lukewarm.

2. Scoop squash and place in large bowl. Remove peel from onions; remove soft garlic from skins and add to squash. Using a blender, puree vegetables together. Pour into large Dutch oven; add broth, cream, and seasonings. Heat over low heat just until warmed through; do not boil.

Nutrition Information: 140 calories, 7g fat, 10mg cholesterol, 250mg sodium, 22g carbohydrate, 3g fiber, 2g protein

Exchanges: 1.5 Carbohydrate, 0 Protein, 1 Fat

Best Ever Vegetable Soup

Makes 6 servings.

2 tablespoons olive oil

1 large onion, chopped

2 cups celery, sliced

2 cups carrots, sliced

2 cloves garlic, minced

2 cups diced potatoes (cut into 1-inch pieces)

4 cups organic low sodium vegetable broth

1 (5.5 oz.) can low-sodium V-8 juice

1 (14.5 oz.) can petite diced tomatoes

2 bay leaves

½ teaspoon each salt and fresh ground black pepper

1 tablespoon Worcestershire sauce

1 ½ cups fresh (or frozen) green beans

1 cup fresh (or frozen) corn kernels

¼ cup fresh chopped parsley

1. In large Dutch oven, heat olive oil over medium heat. Add onion and cook until translucent. Add celery, carrots, and garlic; cook over low heat for 5 minutes or until vegetables begin to soften.

2. Stir in potatoes, vegetable broth, V-8 juice, tomatoes, bay leaves, salt, pepper, and Worcestershire sauce. Bring to boil; then reduce heat and simmer for 20 minutes.

3. Add green beans and corn and cover; simmer soup mixture for an additional 30 minutes. Remove from heat; stir in parsley and serve.

Nutrition Information: 180 calories, 5g fat, 0mg cholesterol, 410mg sodium, 30g carbohydrate, 7g fiber, 5g protein

Exchanges: 2 Carbohydrate, 0.5 Protein, 1 Fat

Boost your veggie consumption! Each vegetable carries its own unique flavor profile and nutritional makeup. Vegetables are a must for anti-inflammatory living!

Crock-Pot Posole

Makes 6 servings.

2 (15 oz.) cans white hominy, drained

2 (10 oz.) cans green enchilada sauce*

1 large onion, chopped

2 cloves garlic, minced

2 teaspoons cumin

½ teaspoon fresh ground black pepper

3 cups low-sodium organic chicken broth

1 ½ pounds pork loin roast

Optional Toppings: chopped cilantro, lime wedges, light sour cream

*Purchase gluten-free enchilada sauce to ensure gluten-free meal.

1. In a large Crock-Pot, stir together hominy, enchilada sauce, onion, garlic, cumin, black pepper, and chicken broth. Add pork, fat side up, and spoon hominy mixture over top. Cook on low for 8-9 hours.

2. Remove pork from crockpot, discard fat, and shred; return to hominy mixture. Serve with desired toppings.

Nutrition Information: 290 calories, 7g fat, 60mg cholesterol, 1170mg sodium, 29g carbohydrate, 4g fiber, 26g protein

Exchanges: 2 Carbohydrate, 3.5 Protein, 1.5 Fat

Cumin has powerful AI properties and is used around the world for its distinctive, warm aroma and flavor. In some countries it is a commonly used treatment for digestive issues.

Hearty Lentil Soup

Makes 8 servings.

2 celery ribs, thinly sliced

1 medium onion, chopped

1 garlic clove, minced

2 tablespoons olive oil

6 cups water

1 (28 oz.) can diced tomatoes

¾ cup dry lentils, rinsed

¾ cup pearl barley

1 tablespoon Better than Boullion
  Vegetable Base

½ teaspoon dried oregano

¼ teaspoon fresh ground black pepper

1 cup carrots, thinly sliced

Optional: 1 cup reduced-fat Swiss
  cheese shreds

1. In a large Dutch oven, sauté celery, onion, and garlic in olive oil until tender. Add water, tomatoes (with liquid), lentils, barley, bouillon, oregano, and pepper; bring to a boil. Reduce heat; cover and simmer for 40 minutes or until lentils and barley are almost tender.

2. Add carrots; simmer for an additional 30 minutes.

3. Sprinkle each serving with cheese, if desired.

Nutrition Information: 220 calories, 4g fat, 0mg cholesterol, 470mg sodium, 37g carbohydrate, 7g fiber, 8g protein

Exchanges: 2.5 Carbohydrate, 1 Protein, 1 Fat

Lentils are small but mighty members of the legume family. These little legumes lead the pack for dietary fiber content, and are rich sources of folate, magnesium, and iron. Lentils are also excellent blood sugar stabilizers and are celebrated for their heart-healthy benefits.

Papa's Chili

Makes 8 servings.

2 pounds 96% lean ground beef

2 onions, chopped

3 cloves garlic, chopped

3 tablespoons chili powder

1 tablespoon oregano

1 teaspoon ground cumin

3 tablespoons flour

½ teaspoon salt

1 teaspoon fresh ground black pepper

1 (10 oz.) can diced tomatoes & green chilies

1 (8 oz.) can tomato sauce

2 (15 oz.) cans pinto beans, rinsed & drained

1. In large Dutch oven, brown ground beef; drain well.

2. Add onions and garlic to meat and cook over low heat until translucent.

3. Mix together chili powder, oregano, cumin, flour, salt, and black pepper and stir into meat. Add 1 quart of water, diced tomatoes and green chilies, tomato sauce, and pinto beans. Simmer for 1-2 hours, adding more water as needed.

Nutrition Information: 300 calories, 7g fat, 70mg cholesterol, 680mg sodium, 32g carbohydrate, 7g fiber, 29g protein

Exchanges: 2 Carbohydrate, 4 Protein, 1.5 Fat

Chili powder is an AI booster that adds vibrancy to almost anything—try sprinkled on melon or as an addition to your favorite chocolate recipes.

Slow Cooker Beef Stew

Makes 8 servings.

1 tablespoon all-purpose flour

1 teaspoon each of celery salt and fresh ground black pepper

2 pounds round steak, trimmed of all visible fat, cut into 1-inch pieces

1 tablespoon canola oil

8 large carrots, peeled and cut into 1-inch pieces

1 pound small red potatoes, quartered

1 (8 oz.) package sliced fresh mushrooms

2 garlic cloves, minced

1 cup diced onion

1 (14.5 oz.) can diced tomatoes

1 (6 oz.) can tomato paste

1 cup low-sodium organic beef broth

½ cup dry red wine

2 tablespoons Worcestershire sauce

1 cup frozen green peas

1. In large bowl, mix together flour and seasonings. Add beef, and toss in flour mixture. In large skillet, heat canola oil over medium heat. Add meat and cook, stirring as needed, until browned.

2. Place beef and vegetables into slow cooker. Add tomatoes, tomato paste, beef broth, wine, and Worcestershire sauce. Cover and cook on low for 6 to 8 hours. Add green peas during last 30 minutes of cooking time.

Nutrition Information: 320 calories, 9g fat, 70mg cholesterol, 500mg sodium, 28g carbohydrate, 6g fiber, 30g protein

Exchanges: 2 Carbohydrate, 4 Protein, 2 Fat

Canola oil is the richest cooking oil source of alpha-linolenic acid, an anti-inflammatory fat linked to improving heart health. For maximum AI benefit, use expeller-pressed canola oil.

Slow Cooker Split Pea Soup

Makes 8 servings.

2 cups (approximately 1 lb.) dried split peas

7 cups water

2 bay leaves

1 cup chopped onions

1 ½ cups peeled and sliced carrots

1 cup chopped celery (include some leafy tops)

2 cups diced potatoes

1 teaspoon salt

¼ teaspoon fresh ground black pepper

Optional: 1 cup diced low-sodium lean ham

1. Place dried peas in slow cooker. Cover with water. Stir in bay leaves, onion, carrots, celery, potatoes, salt, and pepper.

2. Cover and cook on low for 8 hours until peas are tender.

* You may add diced ham with other ingredients before cooking, if desired.

Nutrition Information: 220 calories, 0.5g fat, 0mg cholesterol, 330mg sodium, 42g carbohydrates, 15g fiber, 13g protein

Exchanges: 3 Carbohydrate, 2 Protein, 0 Fat

It's not easy being green! Green peas have prominent antioxidant and anti-inflammatory properties. To add flavor and additional AI benefits, try adding ¹/₂ teaspoon of cardamom to this recipe!

Slow Cooker Chicken Tortilla Soup

Makes 6 servings.

1 can (15 oz.) unsalted, petite diced tomatoes

1 can (10 oz.) red enchilada sauce*

1 can (4 oz.) diced green chilies

1 can (14.5 oz.) black beans, drained & rinsed

1 (10 oz.) bag frozen corn kernels

1 medium onion, finely chopped

2 cloves garlic, minced

1 can (32 oz.) low-sodium chicken broth

1 teaspoon each ground cumin, chili powder, and Mexican oregano

½ teaspoon fresh ground black pepper

4 (approximately 4 oz. each) boneless, skinless chicken breast halves

2 limes, juiced

Optional toppings: fresh cilantro, tortilla chips, shredded cheese, sour cream, diced avocado

*Purchase gluten-free enchilada sauce to ensure a gluten-free meal.

1. Combine all ingredients, except for the lime juice and optional toppings, in a slow cooker. Cook on low setting for 6-8 hours.

2. Remove chicken, shred into bite-sized pieces, and return to soup. Stir in lime juice.

3. Serve with cilantro, tortilla chips, cheese, sour cream, and avocado if desired.

Nutrition Information: 270 calories, 3g fat, 40mg cholesterol, 600mg sodium, 35g carbohydrate, 7g fiber, 26g protein

Exchanges: 2.5 Carbohydrate, 3.5 Protein, 0.5 Fat

Did you know adding citrus juice and fresh ground black pepper will greatly boost the AI benefit of any recipe?

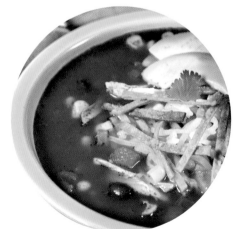

Slow Cooker Chicken Tortilla Soup

Sweet Potato & Black Bean Chili

Makes 8 servings.

2 pounds sweet potatoes, peeled and cut
    into 1-inch cubes

½ teaspoon ground, dried chipotle pepper

½ teaspoon salt

2 tablespoons olive oil, divided

1 onion, diced

4 cloves garlic, minced

1 red bell pepper, diced

1 jalapeño pepper, diced

2 tablespoons ancho chile powder

1 tablespoon ground cumin

¼ teaspoon dried oregano

1 (28 oz.) can diced tomatoes

1 cup water, or more as needed

2 (15 oz.) cans black beans, rinsed
    and drained

1 pinch cayenne pepper

Optional: sour cream and chopped fresh
    cilantro for garnish

1. Preheat oven to 400 degrees.

2. Combine sweet potatoes, chipotle pepper, ½ teaspoon of salt, and 1 tablespoon olive oil in a large bowl and toss to coat. Spread sweet potatoes on baking sheet in a single layer.

3. Roast sweet potatoes in oven about 10 to 15 minutes or until brown; set aside.

4. In large Dutch oven, add remaining 1 tablespoon of olive oil, onion, garlic, red bell pepper, jalapeño pepper, ancho chile powder, cumin, and dried oregano. Cook over medium heat until onion is softened, about 5 minutes, stirring often.

5. Pour tomatoes and water into the onion mixture and bring to a simmer. Reduce heat to low and simmer for 30 minutes.

6. Stir black beans and sweet potatoes into the onion-tomato mixture. Add more water if mixture is too thick. Simmer until heated through, about 15 minutes. Season with salt and cayenne pepper to taste. Serve topped with sour cream and cilantro, if desired.

Nutrition Information: 300 calories, 4g fat, 0mg cholesterol, 600mg sodium, 55g carbohydrate, 13g fiber, 11g protein

Exchanges: 3.5 Carbohydrate, 1.5 Protein, 1 Fat

Black beans are a super source of anthocyanins, and are a great source of iron, B vitamins, and quercitin. A delicious high-fiber food loaded with AI goodness!

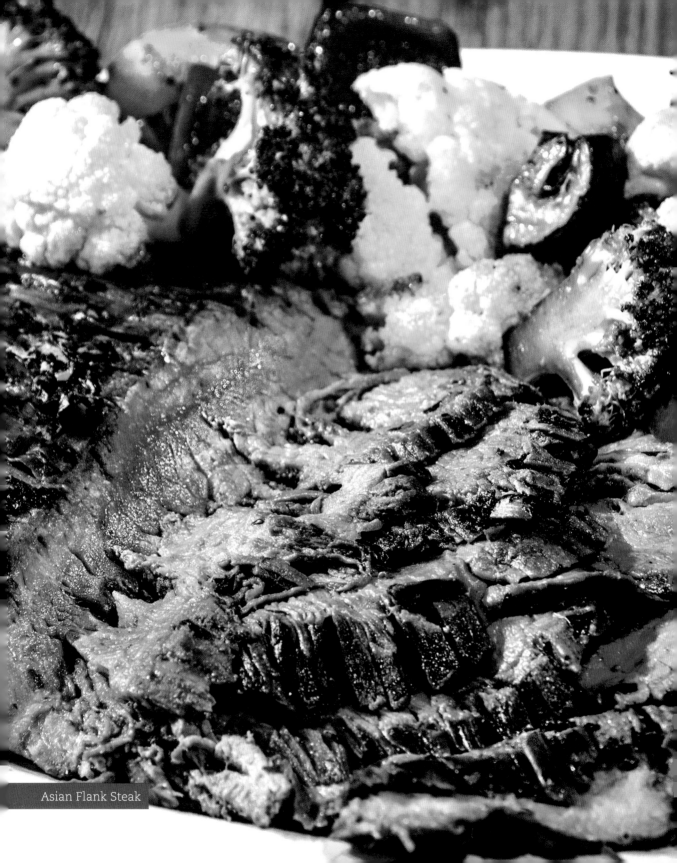
Asian Flank Steak

Asian Flank Steak

Makes 4 servings.

Ingredients:

¼ cup low-sodium tamari sauce

3 tablespoons Worcestershire sauce

2 tablespoons fresh pineapple juice

2 tablespoons chopped fresh cilantro

1 tablespoon minced fresh ginger

1 ¼ pound flank steak, trimmed

Directions:

1. In 13 × 9-inch baking dish, whisk together tamari sauce, Worcestershire sauce, pineapple juice, cilantro, and ginger.

2. Add steak and turn to coat. Let stand 1 hour at room temperature or cover and refrigerate overnight, turning occasionally.

3. Preheat grill to medium heat. Drain marinade into small saucepan and bring to boil; reduce heat and simmer for 2 to 3 minutes to reduce slightly. Grill steak about 5 to 7 minutes per side to desired degree of doneness.

4. Transfer steak to cutting board and let stand for 10 minutes to rest. Thinly slice steak across the grain. Serve with cooked marinade, if desired.

Nutrition Information: 220 calories, 8g fat, 90mg cholesterol, 740mg sodium, 5g carbohydrate, 0g fiber, 31g protein

Exchanges: 0 Carbohydrate, 4.5 Protein, 1.5 Fat

Tamari sauce is the dark, smoky, low-sodium cousin to soy sauce. Like soy sauce, tamari has probiotic properties which can reduce gut inflammation and improve overall immune function.

Beef Tenderloin with Blue Cheese & Mushrooms

Makes 12 servings.

1 pound fresh mushrooms, sliced

1 cup green onions, chopped

1 tablespoon olive oil

¼ cup fresh parsley, chopped

1 (approximately 4 lbs.) beef tenderloin, trimmed

½ teaspoon each seasoned salt & lemon pepper

2 ounces crumbled blue cheese

½ cup red wine vinegar and oil dressing

¼ cup crushed black peppercorns

1. Sauté sliced mushrooms and green onions in olive oil in a large skillet until tender. Stir in parsley; set aside.

2. Split tenderloin length-wise to within ¼ inch of the tenderloin's edge, leaving one long side connected. Sprinkle with seasoned salt and lemon pepper.

3. Spoon mushroom mixture into opening of tenderloin; sprinkle with blue cheese. Fold top side over stuffing and tie securely with heavy string at 2-inch intervals. Place tenderloin in a large, shallow dish. Pour dressing over tenderloin; cover and refrigerate 8 hours, basting with marinade occasionally.

4. Remove tenderloin from dish and discard marinade. Roll tenderloin in crushed peppercorns on waxed paper and place in oven-proof baking dish.

5. Roast in 425-degree oven for 35-40 minutes for medium rare. Remove tenderloin from oven when meat thermometer registers 135 degrees and place on a carving board. Tent loosely with aluminum foil. Let stand 15 minutes. Temperature will continue to rise approximately 10 degrees to reach 145 degrees for medium rare. For medium, cook tenderloin to an internal temperature of 150 degrees and follow same instructions before slicing to serve.

Nutrition Information: 300 calories, 14g fat, 120mg cholesterol, 280mg sodium, 2g carbohydrate, 1g fiber, 39g protein

Exchanges: 0 Carbohydrate, 5.5 Protein, 3 Fat

Beef tenderloin is a very lean cut of meat and is a delicious source of iron, zinc, and folic acid, which are important nutrients for building a strong, healthy body!

Beef

Mexican Shredded Beef (Salpicon) with Serrano Salsa

Makes 12 servings.

4 pounds beef rump roast

1 tablespoon chili powder

1 teaspoon each fresh oregano, cumin, salt, and fresh ground black pepper

1 sweet onion, chopped

2 (10 oz.) cans tomatoes with green chilies

1 cup low-sodium beef broth

1 (4 oz.) can diced green chilies

1 cup water

1. In small bowl, mix together chili powder, oregano, cumin, salt, and pepper. Rub mixture evenly over roast and place in large Dutch oven.

2. Add onion, tomatoes with green chilies, broth, green chilies, and water. Cover tightly and place in oven; bake at 250 degrees for 8-10 hours.

3. Carefully remove roast from pan and let cool slightly. Trim any remaining visible fat; shred meat, using two forks to pull apart, and stir desired amount of pan drippings and tomato mixture into shredded beef.

4. Stir in Serrano-Cilantro Salsa. Place in refrigerator and serve cold, or can be warmed and served on 'street taco' sized corn tortillas.

Serrano-Cilantro Salsa

10 serrano peppers, stemmed and seeded

½ cup diced onion

3 garlic cloves, coarsely chopped

1 tablespoon canola oil

½ cup fresh cilantro, chopped

2 tablespoons fresh lime juice

½ teaspoon salt

¼ teaspoon ground cumin

1. Heat oil in a medium skillet over medium-high heat, stirring occasionally; cook peppers, onion, and garlic for 5-7 minutes, stirring occasionally. Remove from heat, and cool slightly.

2. Process pepper mixture, remaining ingredients, and ½ cup water in a blender until smooth.

Nutrition Information (without tortilla): 290 calories, 13g fat, 150mg cholesterol, 400mg sodium, 7g carbohydrate, 1g fiber, 34g protein

Exchanges: 0.5 Carbohydrate, 5 Protein, 2.5 Fat

Beef

Mushroom-Topped Hamburger Steak on Toasted Baguette

Makes 4 servings.

1 pound 96% lean ground beef

¼ teaspoon fresh ground black pepper

1 tablespoon butter

1 tablespoon olive oil

2 tablespoons onion, thinly sliced

2 tablespoons red bell pepper, cut into thin strips

1 cup fresh mushrooms, cleaned and sliced

½ cup low-sodium beef broth

¼ cup yellow mustard

1 tablespoon Worcestershire sauce

4 (½-inch) slices of whole grain baguette, toasted

1. Shape ground beef into 4 patties about ½ inch thick; season with pepper. Cook patties in a large skillet over medium heat for 5-7 minutes on each side. Remove from skillet and set aside.

2. In same skillet, heat butter and olive oil. Sauté onion, red bell pepper, and mushrooms until tender. Stir in beef broth, mustard, and Worcestershire sauce; bring to a boil; then reduce heat to low simmer. Return steaks to skillet and simmer for 10 minutes, turning once.

3. Place steaks on toasted baguette slices and top with mushroom sauce.

Nutrition Information: 260 calories, 12g fat, 65mg cholesterol, 500mg sodium, 13g carbohydrate, 2g fiber, 27g protein

Exchanges: 1 Carbohydrate, 4 Protein, 2.5 Fat

Mustard: more than just a pretty taste. Mustard seeds are high in selenium, magnesium, and omega-3 fatty acids, giving mustard its anti-inflammatory properties.

Beer-Braised Beef

Makes 12 servings.

4 pounds beef eye of round roast, trimmed of all fat and cut into 1-inch cubes

2 tablespoons flour

2 tablespoons canola oil

2 cups water

2 tablespoons low-sodium beef bouillon granules

4 tablespoons dried onion flakes

2 teaspoons onion powder

½ teaspoon fresh ground black pepper

12 ounces dark beer

1 tablespoon fresh parsley, chopped

1 teaspoon fresh thyme, chopped

Optional: 3 cups cooked brown rice

1. Toss beef cubes in flour, shake off any excess, and brown in canola oil in large skillet over medium heat. Lift meat from skillet and place in 3-quart casserole dish; set aside.

2. Drain fat from skillet, add water, and bring to boil. Carefully stir in beef bouillon granules, onion flakes, onion powder, black pepper, and beer. Pour over meat and sprinkle with parsley and thyme. Cook, covered, at 300 degrees for two hours.

3. Serve meat over cooked rice, if desired.

Nutrition Information: 310 calories, 17g fat, 105mg cholesterol, 160mg sodium, 4g carbohydrate, 0g fiber, 33g protein

Exchanges: 0.5 Carbohydrate, 4 Protein, 3.5 Fat

Lean beef CAN play a part in your healthy diet. Per ounce, beef is higher in protein, B vitamins, iron, and monounsaturated fatty acids than chicken! Choose lean cuts such as sirloin, top-round, or extra lean ground beef.

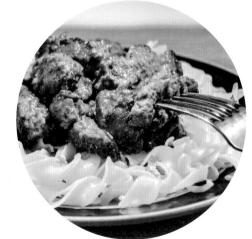

Beer-Braised Beef

One-Pot Spaghetti

Makes 6 servings.

1 pound 96% lean ground beef or ground turkey

1 medium onion, finely chopped

1 green bell pepper, finely chopped

1 cup fresh mushrooms, finely chopped

1 cup each shredded carrot and zucchini

1 (8 oz.) can tomato sauce

1 (14.5 oz.) can petit diced tomatoes

2 teaspoons fresh oregano

1 teaspoon garlic salt

½ teaspoon each salt and fresh ground black pepper

1 tablespoon Worcestershire sauce

6 drops hot pepper sauce (or to taste)

2 cups water

8 ounces whole grain spaghetti noodles

1. In large Dutch oven, brown ground beef over medium heat. Add onion, bell pepper, mushrooms, carrot, and zucchini. Cook for 5 minutes, stirring to incorporate vegetables.

2. Add all remaining ingredients, except spaghetti. Simmer mixture over low heat for 5 minutes. Break spaghetti noodles in half and add (uncooked). Cover pot tightly, reduce heat, and simmer on lowest setting for 30 minutes. Uncover and simmer an additional 10 minutes.

Nutrition Information: 280 calories, 4g fat, 40mg cholesterol, 820g sodium, 42g carbohydrate, 8g fiber, 23g protein

Exchanges: 3 Carbohydrate, 3 Protein, 1 Fat

Porcupine Meatballs

Makes 4 servings.

3 cups prepared low-sodium
   marinara sauce

1 ¼ pounds 96% lean ground beef

1 egg, slightly beaten

⅓ cup onion, finely chopped

½ teaspoon celery salt

⅛ teaspoon ground cayenne pepper

½ teaspoon fresh ground black pepper

2 cloves of garlic, minced

2 teaspoons Worcestershire sauce

2 tablespoons fresh Italian parsley,
   roughly chopped

1 cup brown rice, cooked

Nonstick cooking spray

1. Preheat oven to 375 degrees.
2. In a large glass baking dish, spread ½ cup of marinara sauce; set aide.
3. In a large bowl, combine beef, egg, onion, celery salt, cayenne pepper, black pepper, garlic, Worcestershire sauce, parsley, and rice. Divide and shape the beef mixture into 12 meatballs.
4. In a large skillet, using nonstick cooking spray, brown meatballs in batches until brown on all sides. Place meatballs in baking dish and top with remaining marinara sauce.
5. Cover with foil and bake for 35-40 minutes.

Nutrition Information: 330 calories, 10g fat, 140mg cholesterol, 410mg sodium,
   27g carbohydrate, 3g fiber, 32g protein

Exchanges: 2 Carbohydrate, 4.5 Protein, 2 Fat

Cayenne pepper (also known as capsicum) consumption has been linked to increased metabolism and dilation of blood vessels. Add to your favorite recipes for a spicy punch of anti-inflammatory benefits.

Spinach Beef Casserole

Makes 8 servings.

1 ½ pounds 96% lean ground beef

1 large onion, chopped

1 teaspoon minced garlic

1 cup diced celery

¾ cup grated carrots

2 (14 oz.) cans Italian-style tomatoes

½ teaspoon fresh ground black pepper

1 (8 oz.) package whole grain shell macaroni

1 (10 oz.) package frozen spinach, thawed and squeezed dry

½ cup grated Parmesan cheese

1. Preheat oven to 350 degrees.

2. Place ground beef in large skillet; brown over medium heat and drain well. Add onion, garlic, celery, and carrots; cook, stirring occasionally, until onion is translucent.

3. Add tomatoes, salt, and pepper. Reduce heat, cover, and simmer for 30 minutes, stirring occasionally.

4. Cook macaroni according to package directions; drain well.

5. Combine meat mixture, macaroni, and spinach; mix well. Pour into 9 × 13-inch baking dish. Cover with foil and bake at 350 degrees for 20 minutes. Uncover and sprinkle with cheese. Bake an additional 5 minutes.

Nutrition Information: 300 calories, 6g fat, 50mg cholesterol, 420mg sodium, 37g carbohydrate, 5g fiber, 26g protein

Exchanges: 2.5 Carbohydrate, 4 Protein, 1 Fat

Lycopene is found in tomatoes, pink grapefruit, and watermelon. Research suggests this compound may promote bone health and have protective properties against heart disease and prostate cancer. Unlike most nutrients, lycopene intensifies during the cooking process; the best sources include tomato paste, tomato sauce, and ketchup.

Spaghetti Squash Bake

Makes 6 servings.

1 large spaghetti squash

1 teaspoon olive oil

1 pound lean ground beef or ground turkey

2 cups organic spaghetti sauce

1 cup part-skim ricotta cheese

1 egg, slightly beaten

1 cup part-skim shredded mozzarella cheese, divided

½ teaspoon fresh oregano

5 fresh basil leaves, chiffonade

½ teaspoon each garlic salt & fresh ground black pepper

1. Preheat oven to 350 degrees.

2. Cut spaghetti squash in half lengthwise; rub cut surface with olive oil.

3. Place flesh side down on baking dish and cook for 30-40 minutes until tender. (Time saver tip: squash can be prepared a day before.) Allow squash to cool slightly, then rake out spaghetti strands with a fork. Place in a colander to drain.

4. While squash is draining, prepare sauce: In a large oven-proof skillet, brown meat. Drain off any excess fat and add spaghetti sauce. Carefully stir in squash.

5. In small bowl, mix ricotta cheese, egg, ½ cup of mozzarella cheese, oregano, basil, garlic salt, and pepper. Gently fold cheese mixture until loosely incorporated into the squash, meat, and sauce mixture.

6. Sprinkle remaining mozzarella cheese on top and place in oven. Bake for 30 minutes or until bubbly.

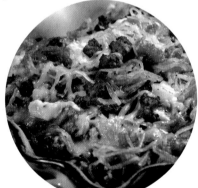

Nutrition Information: 330 calories, 13g fat, 110mg cholesterol, 840mg sodium, 24g carbohydrate, 5g fiber, 30g protein

Exchanges: 1.5 Carbohydrate, 4 Protein, 2.5 Fat

Spaghetti Squash Bake

Spaghetti squash can be microwaved. Poke holes in squash with ice pick or knife tip and cook on high for 10-12 minutes, stopping to turn squash every 3 minutes. Cut in half and allow cooling slightly before raking spaghetti strands with fork.

Beef

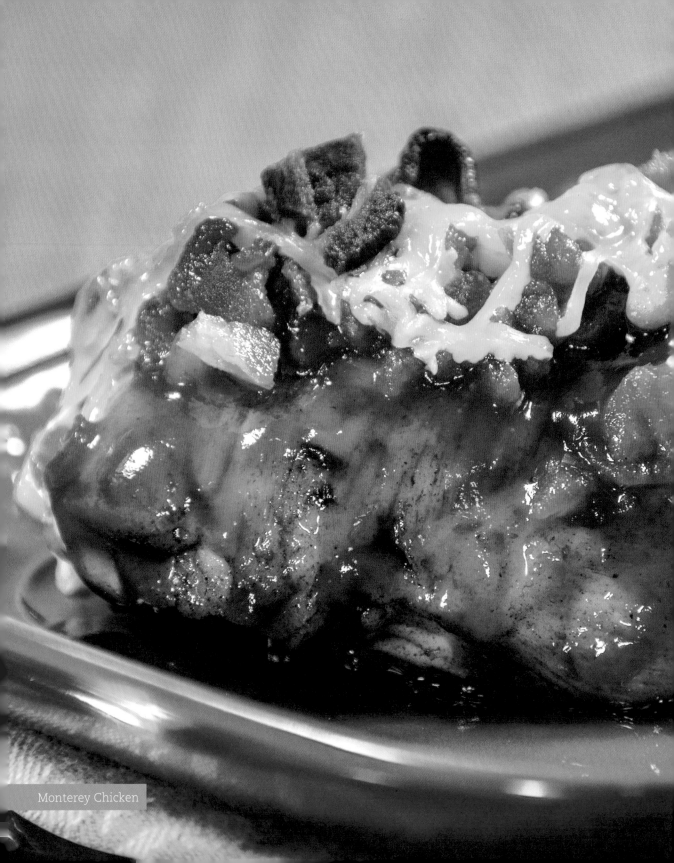

Monterey Chicken

Monterey Chicken

Makes 4 servings.

Ingredients:

4 (approximately 4 oz. each) boneless skinless chicken breasts

½ teaspoon each salt and fresh ground black pepper

1 teaspoon canola oil

¼ cup barbecue sauce

1 (14 oz.) can diced tomatoes with green chilies

1 cup reduced-fat Cheddar cheese shreds

Optional: 2 slices bacon, fried and crumbled

Directions:

1. Preheat oven to 350 degrees.

2. Pat chicken breasts dry and season with salt and pepper.

3. Spray oven-proof skillet with oil; heat over medium-high heat. Add chicken breasts and brown evenly on both sides. Top each chicken breast with 1 tablespoon of barbecue sauce. Spoon evenly with tomatoes and green chilies, and top with cheese shreds and bacon crumbles, if desired.

4. Place in oven and bake for 20 minutes or until cheese melts and chicken is cooked through.

Nutrition Information: 270 calories, 10g fat, 85mg cholesterol, 1110mg sodium, 12g carbohydrate, 1g fiber, 32g protein

Exchanges: 1 Carbohydrate, 4.5 Protein, 2 Fat

30-Minute Chicken Marsala

Makes 4 servings.

4 (approximately 4 oz. each) boneless skinless chicken breast halves

½ teaspoon salt

½ teaspoon fresh cracked black pepper

2 tablespoons olive oil

8 ounces assorted mushrooms, trimmed and sliced

2 shallots, sliced

¾ cup organic low-sodium chicken broth

½ cup Marsala wine

1 tablespoon capers

1 tablespoon chopped parsley

1. Place chicken breasts between 2 pieces of heavy-duty plastic wrap and flatten with meat mallet to ¼-inch thickness. Pat dry on paper towels, then sprinkle with salt and pepper.

2. Heat olive oil in large nonstick skillet over medium-high heat; add chicken and brown 3 to 4 minutes on each side or until golden brown. Remove chicken from skillet; set aside.

3. Add mushrooms and shallots to same skillet; sauté 3 minutes or until tender. Add broth and Marsala to skillet to deglaze pan. Bring mixture to a boil; add capers; reduce heat to medium and cook, stirring occasionally, for 5 minutes or until sauce is slightly reduced. Return chicken to skillet and cook 1 to 2 minutes or until thoroughly heated.

4. Transfer chicken to a serving platter; spoon mushroom mixture over chicken and sprinkle with parsley before serving.

Nutrition Information: 250 calories, 10g fat, 65mg cholesterol, 620mg sodium, 6g carbohydrate, 1g fiber, 25g protein

Exchanges: 0.5 Carbohydrate, 3.5 Protein, 2 Fat

Marsala is a fortified wine extracted from grapes grown in the west portion of Sicily.

Chicken Involtini

Makes 4 servings.

1 (10 oz. bag) baby spinach

¼ cup low-fat ricotta

4 slices (approximately 1 oz. total) thinly sliced prosciutto

4 (approximately 4 oz. each) boneless skinless chicken breast halves, flattened to 1/4 inch thickness

½ teaspoon fresh ground black pepper

1 tablespoon extra-virgin olive oil

2 cloves garlic, minced

1 (14 oz.) can crushed tomatoes

2 tablespoons salted capers, drained & chopped

¼ cup grated Parmesan cheese

2 cups whole grain angel hair pasta, cooked

1. Preheat oven to 400 degrees.

2. Place spinach in a large bowl. Cover with boiling water; let sit for 30 seconds. Pour into colander; drain well and squeeze out excess liquid. Chop and place back in bowl. Stir in ricotta and set aside.

3. Tear sheet of wax paper and place on cutting board. Place one slice of prosciutto on wax paper. Top with flattened chicken breast and sprinkle with black pepper. Place ¼ of spinach mixture on top of chicken and roll to enclose. Use a toothpick to secure. Repeat with remaining prosciutto, chicken and spinach mixture to make 4 chicken rolls.

4. Heat olive oil in large, oven-proof skillet over medium heat. Place chicken rolls in skillet and brown for 3 to 5 minutes on each side. Remove from skillet and keep warm.

5. To same skillet, add garlic and cook over low heat for 2 minutes. Add tomatoes, ½ cup water, and capers and bring to a low simmer. Add chicken rolls and spoon tomato mixture over tops. Place skillet into oven and bake for 15-20 minutes or until chicken is cooked through.

6. Remove from oven and top with cheese. Return to oven and cook for 3-5 minutes or until cheese is brown and crunchy.

7. Serve one chicken roll over ½ cup of pasta.

Nutrition Information: 350 calories, 11g fat, 80mg cholesterol, 770 mg sodium, 30g carbohydrate, 7g fiber, 37g protein

Exchanges: 2 Carbohydrate, 5 Protein, 2 Fat

Hatch Green Chile Chicken & Rice

Makes 4 servings.

4 (approximately 4 oz. each) boneless skinless chicken breast halves

½ teaspoon each salt and fresh ground black pepper

1 tablespoon canola oil

1 large onion, chopped

2 garlic cloves, minced

1 ½ cups organic low-sodium chicken broth

½ cup diced fresh (or 4 oz. can) roasted Hatch green chilies

½ cup salsa

1 cup uncooked brown rice

1 tomato, sliced into 4 slices

1 small avocado, sliced into 8 slices

½ cup reduced-fat cheddar cheese shreds

1. Sprinkle chicken breasts evenly with salt and pepper. Heat oil in large skillet over medium high heat; brown chicken breasts for 3 minutes on each side in oil. Transfer to platter and set aside. In same skillet, add onion and garlic and continue to cook 2 to 3 minutes over low heat, stirring constantly.

2. Add chicken broth, Hatch green chilies, salsa, and rice to onion mixture. Bring to simmer and place chicken breasts on top. Cover tightly and cook over low heat for 20-30 minutes.

3. Remove from heat and let sit for 5 minutes until all liquid is absorbed. Place slice of tomato and 2 slices of avocado on top of each chicken breast. Sprinkle with cheese and serve.

Nutrition Information: 410 calories, 18g fat, 75mg cholesterol, 760mg sodium, 32g carbohydrate, 6g fiber, 33g protein

Exchanges: 2 Carbohydrate, 5 Protein, 4 Fat

Italian Turkey Meatball Packets

Makes 4 servings.

½ cup whole grain bread crumbs

¼ cup grated Parmesan cheese

1 clove garlic, minced

½ cup finely chopped onion

2 tablespoons each chopped fresh basil and fresh Italian parsley

2 tablespoons 1% milk

1 tablespoon tomato paste

½ teaspoon each salt and fresh ground black pepper

1 egg, slightly beaten

1 pound extra lean ground turkey

½ medium sweet onion, cut into thin strips

½ medium green bell pepper, cut into thin strips

½ medium red bell pepper, cut into thin strips

1 cup organic marinara sauce

4 tablespoons grated Parmesan cheese

1. In medium bowl, combine breadcrumbs, cheese, garlic, onion, herbs, milk, tomato paste, salt, pepper, and egg. Stir to blend well.

2. Add ground turkey, using fingers to gently mix all ingredients. Shape into eight 1-inch balls and place 2 inches apart on nonstick baking sheet with sides and bake until cooked through, about 10 minutes.

3. Tear off 4 18 × 12-inch sheets of aluminum foil; spray 1 side of each sheet with cooking spray.

4. Place 2 meatballs in center of greased side of each foil sheet. Top meatballs evenly with onions, bell peppers and ¼ cup marinara sauce.

5. Bring together 2 sides of each foil sheet over ingredients, and double fold with about 1-inch-wide folds. Double fold each end to form a packet, leaving room for heat circulation inside packet. Place packets on baking sheet.

6. Bake at 400 degrees for 30 minutes. Carefully open packets to prevent burns from hot steam. Sprinkle each serving with 1 tablespoon cheese before serving.

If desired, serve meatballs over whole wheat pasta or create an Italian meatball sub by placing meatballs on a toasted roll topped with a slice of mozzarella cheese.

Nutrition Information: 320 calories, 10g fat, 125mg cholesterol, 1010mg sodium, 23g carbohydrate, 3g fiber, 38g protein

Exchanges: 1.5 Carbohydrate, 5.5 Protein, 2 Fat

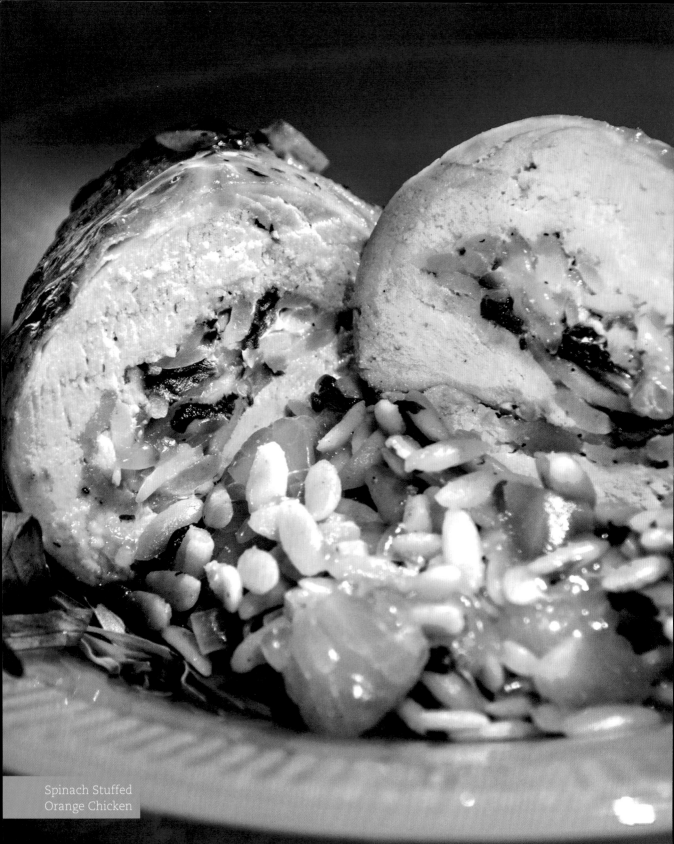

Spinach Stuffed
Orange Chicken

Spinach Stuffed Orange Chicken

Makes 4 servings.

4 (approximately 4 oz. each) boneless skinless chicken breast halves

½ teaspoon seasoned salt

1 tablespoon olive oil

Stuffing:

1 teaspoon olive oil

¼ cup chopped onion

½ cup diced fresh mushrooms

2 cups fresh spinach, coarsely chopped

½ teaspoon minced garlic

1 ½ cups cooked whole wheat orzo

1 (11 oz.) can mandarin oranges, drain and reserve liquid

¼ teaspoon each salt and fresh ground black pepper

Tarragon-Orange Sauce:

½ cup fresh orange juice

½ cup reserved mandarin orange liquid

1 cup organic low-sodium chicken broth

1 tablespoon cornstarch

1 teaspoon fresh tarragon leaves

¼ teaspoon each salt and fresh ground black pepper

1. Preheat oven to 350 degrees.

2. Place chicken breast between 2 pieces of (double thickness) plastic wrap. Pound chicken with flat side of meat mallet until about ¼-inch thick. Repeat with remaining chicken breasts; set aside.

3. To prepare stuffing: In large oven-proof skillet, sauté onion, mushrooms, spinach, and garlic in olive oil. Stir into orzo, add drained mandarin oranges, and season with salt and pepper.

4. Place ¼ cup stuffing mixture down center of each chicken breast. (Reserve remaining orzo mixture in medium bowl to serve with chicken.) Bring ends over stuffing and tuck inside. Roll and secure with wooden picks, if desired. Sprinkle evenly with seasoned salt.

5. Wipe skillet clean; add one tablespoon olive oil and brown chicken on both sides, turning carefully to not lose stuffing. Remove from skillet and set aside.

6. In small bowl, whisk together sauce ingredients. Add sauce to same skillet and bring to a boil over medium-high heat. Cook 3 to 5 minutes or until sauce is thickened, stirring constantly. Return chicken to skillet and ladle with sauce.

7. Bake, uncovered, for 30 minutes or until chicken is tender. Heat remaining orzo mixture and serve with chicken.

Nutrition Information: 320 calories, 8g fat, 65mg cholesterol, 680mg sodium, 35g carbohydrate, 2g fiber, 28g protein

Exchanges: 2 Carbohydrate, 4 Protein, 1.5 Fat

Pesto Chicken Skewers

Makes 8 servings.

2 pounds skinless boneless chicken breast, cut into 1-inch cubes

½ cup prepared basil pesto

24 cherry tomatoes

8 wooden skewers

½ teaspoon each sea salt and fresh cracked black pepper

1. Preheat grill to medium.

2. In a large zippered plastic bag, combine the chicken cubes with pesto and marinate for 2 to 4 hours. Soak wooden skewers in water at least 30 minutes.

3. Beginning and ending with chicken, thread chicken and tomatoes onto skewers. Season with salt and pepper. Discard remaining marinade.

4. Place chicken kabobs on grill and cook 3-4 minutes; turn and continue cooking until chicken is cooked through, about 3-4 minutes.

Nutrition Information: 210 calories, 10g fat, 65mg cholesterol, 330mg sodium, 3g carbohydrate, 1g fiber, 25g protein

Exchanges: 0 Carbohydrate, 3.5 Protein, 2 Fat

Braised Chicken with Butternut Squash, Mushrooms & New Potatoes

Makes 4 servings.

2 tablespoons olive oil, divided

4 (approximately 4 oz. each) boneless skinless chicken breast halves

¼ teaspoon salt

½ teaspoon fresh cracked black pepper

1 sweet onion, finely chopped

½ pound of shiitake or button mushrooms, stemmed and quartered

2 cups small new potatoes, cut into wedges

1 butternut squash, peeled, seeded, and cut into ½-inch pieces*

1 tablespoon fresh sage, minced

1 ¾ cups low-sodium, low-fat chicken broth, divided

1-2 teaspoons all-purpose flour

*I like using fresh-cut butternut squash cubes found in the produce section of most supermarkets—saves lots of work!

1. In large skillet, place 1 tablespoon olive oil over medium heat.

2. Pat chicken dry and sprinkle with salt and pepper. Brown on both sides in oil. Remove from skillet and transfer to a plate. Reduce heat to medium.

3. In same skillet, add 1 tablespoon olive oil and sauté onion, mushrooms, and potato wedges until tender, about 5 minutes. Add squash and sage; toss to coat with oil.

4. Return chicken to skillet and add 1 ½ cups chicken broth; bring to a boil, reduce heat to low, cover and simmer until chicken is tender, about 30 minutes.

5. In small bowl, whisk together remaining ¼ cup chicken broth and flour. Add to skillet, mix, and simmer until sauce thickens.

Nutrition Information: 320 calories, 10g fat, 65mg cholesterol, 280mg sodium, 28g carbohydrate, 3g fiber, 29g protein

Exchanges: 2 Carbohydrate, 4 Protein, 2 Fat

Just one cup of butternut squash contains over 400% of your RDA for Vitamin A—a powerful anti-oxidant needed for optimal eye and skin health.

Italian Chicken with Peppers & Olives

Makes 4 servings.

4 (approximately 5 oz. each) skinless bone-in chicken breasts

1 tablespoon olive oil

2 garlic cloves, crushed

2 ounces Kalamata olives (save juice)

6 ounces pepperoncini (save juice)

4 ounces sun-dried tomatoes

2 cups cooked whole wheat angel hair pasta

1. In large Dutch oven, brown chicken in olive oil. Remove chicken from pot, add crushed garlic, and cook for 2 minutes. Add olives, pepperoncini, and sun-dried tomatoes. Add about ½ cup of juice from both olives and pepperoncini to make 1 cup of liquid.

2. Return chicken to pot, cover, and bake at 350 degrees for 1 hour.

3. Serve over whole wheat angel hair pasta.

Nutrition Information: 370 calories, 11g fat, 65mg cholesterol, 1380mg sodium, 39g carbohydrate, 7g fiber, 31g protein

Exchanges: 2.5 Carbohydrate, 4.5 Protein, 2 Fat

Penne Pasta with Spinach, Feta & Grilled Chicken

Makes 4 servings.

4 (approximately 4 oz. each) boneless skinless chicken breast halves

½ teaspoon each sea salt and fresh cracked black pepper

2 cups cooked whole grain pasta

5 large plum tomatoes, seeded and diced

2 cups fresh spinach

4 green onions, chopped

2 tablespoons prepared pesto

2 tablespoons fresh oregano, chopped

2 tablespoons fresh basil, chopped

¼ teaspoon salt

¼ teaspoon fresh cracked black pepper

2 ounces reduced-fat basil-and-tomato crumbled feta cheese

1. Preheat indoor or outdoor grill. Rub chicken with salt and pepper. Grill chicken for 5-7 minutes per side over medium heat. Remove to platter, tent with foil, and set aside.

2. Prepare pasta in a large Dutch oven, according to package directions; drain. Return to Dutch oven.

3. Stir in tomatoes and next 7 ingredients; cook 2 minutes over medium heat.

4. Plate pasta onto 4 plates. Top with thinly sliced grilled chicken breast, sprinkle with cheese, and serve.

Nutrition Information: 420 calories, 12g fat, 65mg cholesterol, 720mg sodium, 42g carbohydrate, 10g fiber, 36g protein

Exchanges: 3 Carbohydrate, 5 Protein, 2 Fat

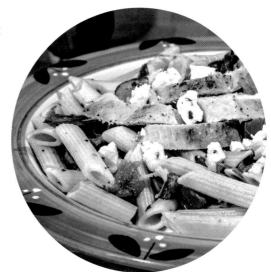

Penne Pasta with Spinach, Feta & Grilled Chicken

Turkey Cheeseburger with Caramelized Onions

Makes 6 servings.

1 large sweet onion

2 tablespoons olive oil, divided

1 (20 oz.) package lean ground turkey breast

1 large egg, lightly beaten

½ teaspoon salt

½ teaspoon fresh ground black pepper

1 teaspoon balsamic vinegar

½ teaspoon fresh rosemary, optional

6 thin slices reduced-fat Swiss cheese

6 whole grain hamburger buns

Optional toppings: lettuce leaves, Dijon mustard, tomato slices

1. Cut ¼ of onion and dice; then cut remaining onion into thin slices and set aside. Heat ½ tablespoon olive oil in large skillet. Sauté diced onion until translucent; set aside.

2. In a medium bowl, gently combine turkey, egg, salt, and pepper with sautéed onion. Shape mixture into 6 patties.

3. Heat 1 tablespoon olive oil in same skillet over medium-high heat; add remaining onion slices and sauté 10 minutes or until onion is tender and golden. Stir in balsamic vinegar and rosemary, if desired. Remove onion mixture from skillet.

4. Add remaining ½ tablespoon olive oil to same skillet and place over medium-high heat. Cook patties 5 minutes on each side or until no longer pink in the center. Place on an aluminum foil-lined baking sheet.

5. Top each patty evenly with onion mixture and 1 cheese slice. Broil 6 inches from heat for 3 minutes or until cheese is lightly browned. Serve on toasted buns with desired toppings.

Nutrition Information: 380 calories, 17g fat, 105mg cholesterol, 500mg sodium, 28g carbohydrate, 3g fiber, 31g protein

Exchanges: 2 Carbohydrate, 4.5 Protein, 3.5 Fat

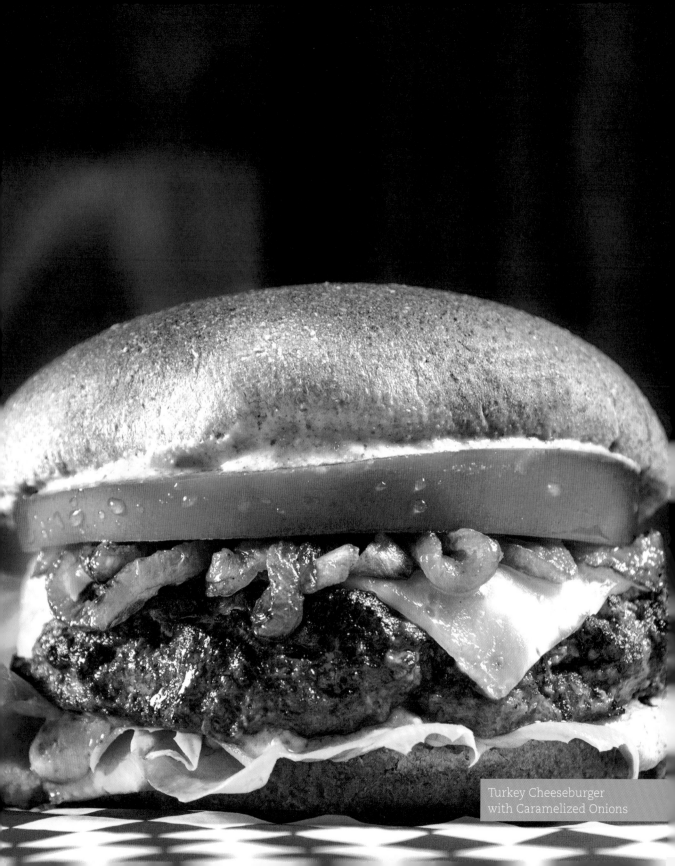

Turkey Cheeseburger
with Caramelized Onions

Mediterranean Chicken Sandwiches

Makes 4 sandwiches.

Grilled chicken:

1 cup low-fat buttermilk

2 teaspoons salt

2 teaspoons curry powder

1 teaspoon each fresh ground black pepper, cumin, and turmeric

4 (approximately 4 oz. each) boneless skinless chicken breast halves

Tzatziki Sauce:

1 large cucumber, peeled and chopped fine

½ small red onion, chopped fine

1 tablespoon light sour cream

1 teaspoon fresh lemon juice

¾ teaspoon celery seeds

1 tablespoon plain Greek yogurt

Bread and Spread:

8 slices whole grain artisan bread

1 tablespoon olive oil

2 tablespoons hummus

4 sprigs fresh dill, chopped

1. Combine buttermilk, salt, curry, black pepper, cumin, and turmeric in a large re-sealable plastic bag. Add chicken to bag, seal, and turn to coat. Chill at least 4 hours or overnight.

2. Prepare grill for medium-high heat. Meanwhile, in medium bowl combine cucumber, red onion, sour cream, lemon juice, celery seeds, and Greek yogurt.

3. Remove chicken from marinade and discard marinade. Grill chicken until cooked through, 5–7 minutes per side.

4. Brush bread on both sides with oil and grill until toasted, about 2 minutes per side; spread with hummus. Layer with chicken breast and tzatziki sauce, sprinkle with fresh dill, and enjoy!

Nutrition Information: 350 calories, 10g fat, 65mg cholesterol, 430mg sodium, 34g carbohydrate, 4g fiber, 31g protein

Exchanges: 2 Carbohydrate, 4.5 Protein, 2 Fat

Orange Marmalade Almond Chicken

Makes 4 servings.

⅓ cup lemon juice

3 tablespoons Dijon mustard

2 garlic cloves, minced

1 tablespoon olive oil

½ teaspoon fresh ground white pepper

4 (approximately 4 oz. each) boneless
   skinless chicken breast halves

1 tablespoon olive oil

2 cups organic low-sodium chicken broth

1 teaspoon cornstarch

1 tablespoon water

3 tablespoons orange marmalade

½ teaspoon each salt and fresh ground
   black pepper

¼ teaspoon dried crushed red pepper

2 tablespoons chopped fresh parsley

¼ cup sliced almonds, toasted

2 cups cooked brown rice

1. Whisk together first 5 ingredients. Reserve ¼ cup for sauce. Pour remaining marinade into plastic zippered bag. Add chicken, chill 1 hour.

2. Remove chicken from marinade; discard marinade; cook chicken in hot oil in a large skillet over medium-high heat 5 minutes on each side. Remove chicken, reserving drippings in skillet.

3. Add reserved ¼ cup marinade mixture and chicken broth to skillet, stirring to loosen browned bits from bottom of skillet.

4. Stir together cornstarch and water; add to broth mixture. Bring to a boil; cook, stirring constantly, 1 minute. Stir in marmalade and next 4 ingredients.

5. Return chicken to skillet and spoon sauce over chicken. Cover and let simmer for 5 minutes over low heat. Sprinkle with parsley and almonds.

6. To serve, place ½ cup brown rice on each plate. Top with chicken breast, drizzle with sauce, and serve.

Nutrition Information: 440 calories, 16g fat, 70mg cholesterol, 690mg sodium,
   45g carbohydrate, 3g fiber, 28g protein

Exchanges: 3 Carbohydrate, 4 Protein, 3 Fat

*Parsley is so much more than a beautiful garnish! It is rich in Vitamin K, a vitamin needed
   for blood clotting. Try a combination of parsley, lemon zest, and fresh minced garlic for a
   delicious calorie-free, anti-inflammatory rub for chicken, beef, and lamb!*

Sherried Chicken with Mushrooms & Artichokes

Makes 6 servings.

6 (approximately 4 oz. each) boneless skinless chicken breast halves

1 teaspoon paprika

½ teaspoon fresh ground black pepper

3 tablespoons olive oil, divided

1 (14 oz.) can artichoke hearts, drained and halved

1 ½ cups fresh mushrooms, quartered

¼ cup sliced green onions

1 tablespoon cornstarch

1 cup organic low-sodium chicken broth

¼ cup dry sherry

1. Preheat oven to 375 degrees.

2. Sprinkle chicken on both sides with paprika and black pepper. Brown chicken in 2 table-spoons olive oil in large skillet over medium-high heat for 2 minutes on each side. Place chicken in 9 × 13-inch baking dish. Arrange artichoke hearts around chicken; set aside.

3. In same skillet, heat remaining olive oil over medium heat. Add mushrooms and green onions and cook, stirring frequently, 4 to 5 minutes. Combine cornstarch, broth, and sherry; add to skillet. Bring to a boil; cook, stirring constantly, for 1 minute. Pour mixture over chicken and artichokes. Cover with aluminum foil and bake for 30 minutes or until chicken is done.

Nutrition Information: 270 calories, 11g fat, 75mg cholesterol, 430mg sodium, 10g carbohydrate, 2g fiber, 26g protein

Exchanges: 0.5 Carbohydrate, 3.5 Protein, 2 Fat

Yogurt Marinated Grilled Chicken

Makes 6 servings.

½ cup plain Greek yogurt

2 minced garlic cloves

2 tablespoons lemon juice

Zest of one lemon

1 tablespoon olive oil

½ teaspoon each of chili powder, ground ginger, cumin, and salt

6 (approximately 4 oz. each) boneless skinless chicken breasts

1. In large bowl, whisk together all ingredients except chicken breasts. Pour ⅔ of yogurt mixture into a plastic zippered bag; add chicken breasts, turning to coat. Place chicken in refrigerator and marinate 8 hours or overnight. Reserve remaining marinade in refrigerator to serve with grilled chicken.

2. Prepare grill, remove chicken from marinade, and cook over medium heat for about 6 to 8 minutes on each side. Discard used marinade.

3. Serve grilled chicken with reserved yogurt sauce, if desired.

Nutrition Information: 170 calories, 7g fat, 65mg cholesterol, 260mg sodium, 2g carbohydrate, 0g fiber, 24g protein

Exchanges: 0 Carbohydrate, 3.5 Protein, 1.5 Fat

A healthy digestive tract is full of healthy, active bacteria. Probiotics, found in yogurt, can support this healthy gut environment.

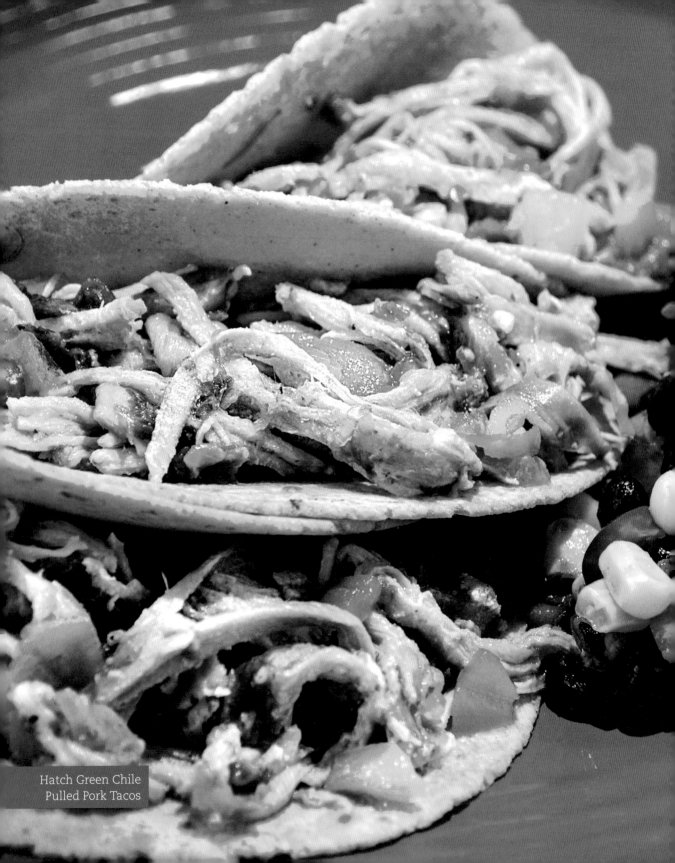
Hatch Green Chile
Pulled Pork Tacos

Hatch Green Chile Pulled Pork Tacos

Makes 12 tacos.

Ingredients:

1 3-pound lean pork tenderloin roast

1 teaspoon Montreal Steak Seasoning

1 teaspoon each ground cumin and garlic salt

½ teaspoon fresh ground black pepper

1 small onion, cut in half and sliced thin

3 mild Hatch green chilies, roasted, skin and seeds removed

½ cup water

½ cup salsa verde

12 corn tortillas

¼ cup chopped fresh cilantro

Directions:

1. Place pork roast, fat side up, in slow cooker. Sprinkle evenly with seasonings. Arrange sliced onion around sides of pork.

2. Lay peppers across top of pork. Add water, cover with lid, and cook on low for 6-8 hours.

3. Remove pork from slow cooker. Carefully remove peppers and onions and reserve. Pour cooking liquid through strainer and reserve. Discard fat from pork and, using two forks, pull meat apart to shred.

4. Place shredded meat back in slow cooker. Slice chilies and add with onions to shredded meat. Stir in salsa verde and about ½ cup of reserved liquid or enough to moisten meat mixture.

5. Serve on corn tortillas; top with cilantro.

Nutrition Information: 210 calories, 8g fat, 60mg cholesterol, 290mg sodium, 13g carbohydrate, 2g fiber, 22g protein

Exchanges: 1 Carbohydrate, 3 Protein, 2.5 Fat

Pork

Foil-Wrapped Mexican Pork Chops

Makes 6 servings.

6 (approximately 4 oz. each) center-cut
  boneless pork chops

½ teaspoon fresh ground black pepper

1 teaspoon chili powder

2 cups chunky salsa

1 (15.25 oz.) can black beans, rinsed
  and drained

1 (10 oz.) package frozen sweet corn

2 cups brown rice, cooked

½ cup low-fat pepper jack cheese
  cheese shreds

1. Tear off 4 large sheets of heavy-duty aluminum foil.

2. Place 1 pork chop in center of each foil sheet. Sprinkle evenly with pepper and chili powder.

3. In a medium bowl, stir together salsa, beans, corn, and rice; spoon evenly over chops.

4. Bring up 2 sides of each foil sheet and double fold together. Fold each end to seal and create package.

5. Place in 350-degree oven for 30 minutes; or grill, covered, over indirect heat for 30-40 minutes or until done. Remove from grill, carefully open packets, sprinkle evenly with cheese, and serve.

Nutrition Information: 420 calories, 13g fat, 65mg cholesterol, 540mg sodium, 43g carbohydrate, 7g fiber, 31g protein

Exchanges: 3 Carbohydrate, 4.5 Protein, 2 Fat

Maple-Glazed Pork Chops

Makes 4 servings.

- 3 tablespoons lightly packed brown sugar
- 2 teaspoons fresh ground black pepper
- ½ teaspoon salt
- 1 teaspoon onion powder
- 1 teaspoon paprika
- 4 (approximately 4 oz. each) center-cut boneless pork chops
- 2 tablespoons pure maple syrup
- 2 tablespoons spicy brown mustard

1. To prepare rub, stir together brown sugar, pepper, salt, onion powder, and paprika in small bowl.

2. Place pork chops in flat baking dish and coat chops with rub mixture on both sides. Cover and place in refrigerator for 4 to 8 hours or overnight. (The longer the chops can sit in the rub, the more intense the flavor!)

3. When ready to grill, prepare glaze by stirring together maple syrup and mustard in small bowl; set aside.

4. Prepare grill. Heat coals to medium-high heat. Place pork chops on grill and cook for 5 to 7 minutes on one side. Turn and cook for another 5 to 7 minutes depending on thickness of chops.

5. Brush chops with maple-mustard glaze and cook for 1 minute. Turn, brush with glaze and cook an additional minute. Remove chops to serving plate and top with remaining glaze, if desired.

Nutrition Information: 300 calories, 7g fat, 105mg cholesterol, 500mg sodium, 17g carbohydrate, 1g fiber, 43g protein

Exchanges: 1 Carbohydrate, 6 Protein, 1 Fat

Pistachio Crusted Pork Tenderloin

Makes 8 servings.

1 2-pound packaged pork tenderloin

1 tablespoon olive oil

1 teaspoon Cavender's Greek Seasoning

1 teaspoon fresh cracked black pepper

⅓ cup crushed pistachios

Optional: ½ cup raspberry chipotle sauce

1. Preheat oven to 375 degrees.

2. Rub pork tenderloin with olive oil. Season with Cavender's and black pepper and roll in crushed pistachios.

3. Place on baking sheet and bake, uncovered, for 30 minutes or until meat thermometer reads 145 degrees. Remove from oven and let pork rest for 5 minutes. Slice into ½-inch slices.

4. Warm raspberry chipotle sauce and serve to accompany pork tenderloin, if desired.

Nutrition Information: 230 calories, 15g fat, 60mg cholesterol, 140mg sodium, 3g carbohydrate, 1g fiber, 22g protein

Exchanges: 0 Carbohydrate, 3 Protein, 3 Fat

Pistachios are rich in mono- and polyunsaturated fatty acids and insoluble fiber, making this little nut the perfect anti-inflammatory snack. Try adding pistachios to salads, baked goods, or yogurt.

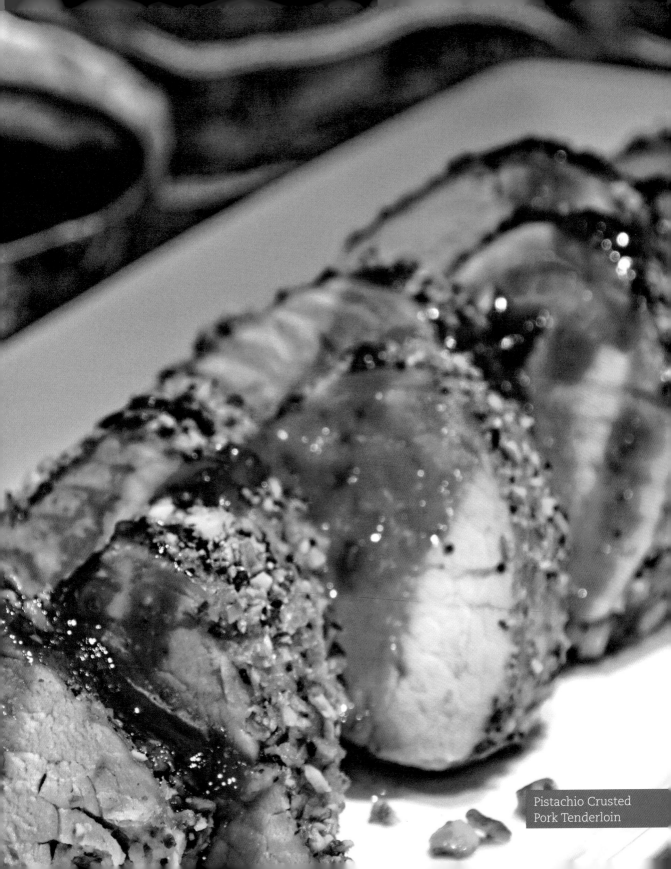

Pistachio Crusted
Pork Tenderloin

Pork, Red Pepper & Snow Pea Stir-Fry with Roasted Cashews

Makes 4 servings.

1 tablespoon dry sherry

2 teaspoons cornstarch

3 tablespoons low-sodium soy sauce, divided

2 teaspoons sesame oil

1 ¾-pound pork loin, trimmed of all fat, cut into ¼-inch strips

1 tablespoon canola oil

1 tablespoon minced fresh ginger

2 cloves garlic, minced

½ teaspoon crushed red pepper flakes

1 red bell pepper, sliced into ¼-inch strips

½ pound snow peas, strings removed

¼ cup cashews, roasted

2 cups steamed brown rice

1. In medium bowl, stir together sherry, cornstarch, and 1 tablespoon soy sauce, then stir in sesame oil. Add pork, stirring to coat well, and let stand 10 minutes.

2. Heat large nonstick skillet or wok over high heat. Add 1 tablespoon canola oil, swirling to coat pan evenly. Stir-fry ginger, garlic, and pepper flakes until fragrant, about 5 seconds. Add bell pepper and stir-fry 2 minutes. Add snow peas and cashews and stir-fry until crisp tender, 1-2 min. Remove from skillet and set aside.

3. To same skillet, add pork and stir-fry, separating strips until browned and barely cooked through, 2-3 minutes. Return vegetables to skillet, add remaining soy sauce, and stir-fry until vegetables are just heated through, about 1 minute. Serve over steamed brown rice.

Nutrition Information: 360 calories, 13g fat, 45mg cholesterol, 500mg sodium, 40g carbohydrate, 4g fiber, 22g protein

Exchanges: 2.5 Carbohydrate, 3 Protein, 2.5 Fat

Roast Pork with Apples & Mushrooms

Makes 10 servings.

1 3-pound boneless pork tenderloin roast

1 teaspoon salt

½ teaspoon fresh ground black pepper

½ teaspoon thyme leaves

1 tablespoon flour

1 tablespoon canola oil

1 large sweet onion, cut into thin wedges

2 apples, cored, peeled, and sliced into quarters

1 (16 oz.) package fresh white button mushrooms, cleaned and quartered

1 cup dry white wine

¼ cup half and half

1. Preheat oven to 325 degrees.

2. Place pork tenderloin roast on large piece of waxed paper. Sprinkle evenly with salt, pepper, and thyme leaves. Lightly rub with flour.

3. In large Dutch oven, heat oil over medium heat. Add roast and brown evenly on all sides; remove and set aside.

4. To same Dutch oven, add onion and cook over medium heat for about 3 minutes. Stir in apples and mushrooms and continue to cook for 5 minutes. Move onions, apples, and mushrooms to sides of pan and return pork to Dutch oven. Pour wine over pork and add about 1 cup of water. Cover with tight-fitting lid and place in oven for 2 ½ to 3 hours.

5. Remove pork and apple-mushroom mixture to serving platter and tent with foil. Reserve pan juices in Dutch oven; place over medium-high heat and reduce liquid by about one-third. Stir in half and half and heat through. Slice pork and plate with serving of apple-mushroom mixture. Top each serving with a generous drizzle of sauce and serve.

Nutrition Information: 210 calories, 6g fat, 75mg cholesterol, 300mg sodium, 7g carbohydrate, 1g fiber, 27g protein

Exchanges: 0.5 Carbohydrate, 4 Protein, 1 Fat

Layers and layers of benefits! Onions, while high in vitamins and minerals, are especially high in the antioxidant quercetin, which plays a significant role in the prevention of atherosclerosis and heart disease.

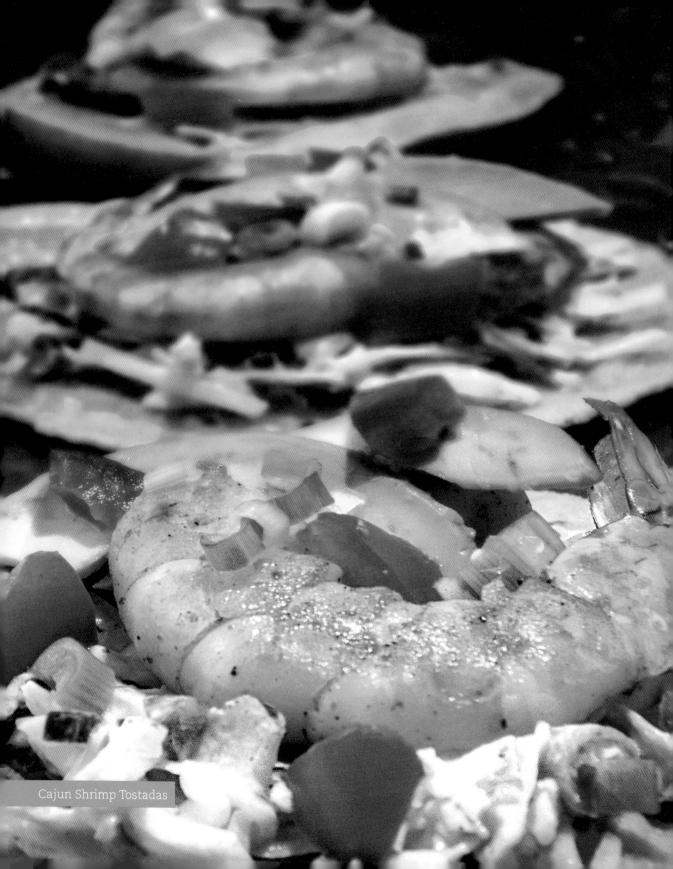

Cajun Shrimp Tostadas

Cajun Shrimp Tostadas

Makes 4 servings.

Ingredients:

4 large corn tortillas

Olive oil cooking spray

24 large shrimp, peeled and deveined

1 teaspoon canola oil

1 ½ teaspoons Cajun seasoning, divided

4 cups shredded coleslaw mix

2 green onions, thinly sliced

¼ cup light sour cream

2 teaspoons fresh lime juice

1 medium tomato, diced

1 avocado, thinly sliced

¼ cup fresh cilantro

Fresh lime wedges

Directions:

1. Spray corn tortillas with cooking spray and place on baking sheet into preheated 400-degree oven for 5 minutes or until crisp; set aside.

2. In medium bowl, toss together shrimp, canola oil, and 1 teaspoon Cajun seasoning. Place shrimp in single layer into hot skillet and sauté for 2 minutes on each side; set aside.

3. In separate bowl, combine coleslaw mix, green onion, sour cream, lime juice, and ½ teaspoon Cajun seasoning.

4. Assemble tostadas by topping with coleslaw blend, tomatoes, shrimp, avocado slices, and cilantro. Serve with lime wedges.

Nutrition Information: 320 calories, 12g fat, 260mg cholesterol, 540mg sodium, 23g carbohydrate, 7g fiber, 31g protein

Exchanges: 1.5 Carbohydrate, 4 Protein, 2 Fat

Shrimp is an unlikely source of the antioxidant selenium and the anti-inflammatory carotenoid, astaxanthin. These two compounds make shrimp a disease-fighting protein powerhouse, weighing in at 18g protein per 3 oz. serving.

Balsamic Grilled Salmon with Spinach & Tomatoes

Makes 4 servings.

4 (approximately 5 oz. each)
   salmon filets

¼ cup light balsamic vinaigrette

½ teaspoon each sea salt and fresh
   cracked black pepper

1 tablespoon olive oil

1 small yellow onion, diced

2 cloves garlic, minced

6 Roma tomatoes, diced

1 (10 oz.) bag of baby spinach

1 tablespoon capers, rinsed & drained

2 cups cooked whole grain angel
   hair pasta

1 lemon, cut into 4 wedges

Seafood

1. Place salmon filets in large plastic zippered bag. Pour vinaigrette over salmon; seal bag and allow filets to marinate in the refrigerator for 30 minutes while you are preparing the other ingredients.

2. Sprinkle salmon with salt and pepper. Place flesh side down on hot grill. Cook 5 minutes; then turn to cook, skin side down, for an additional 5 minutes or until salmon is cooked to desired degree of doneness.

3. While salmon is grilling, heat olive oil in large nonstick skillet. Add onions and garlic; sauté about 5 minutes or until translucent. Stir in tomatoes, spinach, and capers; cook an additional 2 minutes.

4. Carefully remove salmon from grill, leaving skin on grill. Place filets on top of cooked angel hair pasta, and top with spinach mixture. Squeeze with juice from lemon wedge and serve.

Nutrition Information: 410 Calories, 15g fat, 90mg cholesterol, 550mg sodium, 31g carbohydrate, 6g fiber, 38g protein

Exchanges: 2 Carbohydrate, 5.5 Protein, 3 Fat

The American Heart Association recommends eating at least two (3.5 oz) servings of fish each week. Salmon is rich in anti-inflammatory omega-3 fatty acids and has been shown to improve your mood and provide significant cardiovascular protection.

Blackened Fish Tacos

Makes 4 servings (2 tacos each).

4 (approximately 4 oz. each) tilapia filets, cut in half, lengthwise

1 teaspoon blackened seasoning

1 tablespoon canola oil

4 cups shredded coleslaw mix

¼ cup light sour cream

2 teaspoons fresh lime juice

⅛ teaspoon spicy Cajun seasoning

8 6-inch corn tortillas

8 slices avocado

¼ cup fresh cilantro, chopped

Optional: 2 tablespoons fresh jalapeños, finely chopped

Fresh lime wedges

1. Sprinkle tilapia filets with 1 teaspoon blackened seasoning. Place canola oil in large skillet over medium heat; brown tilapia for 3-4 minutes on each side.

2. While cooking tilapia, combine coleslaw mix, sour cream, lime juice, and Cajun seasoning.

3. Heat tortillas and assemble fish tacos by placing one fish filet on each corn tortilla. Top with coleslaw blend, avocado slices, and cilantro. Add jalapeños, if desired. Serve with lime wedges.

Nutrition Information: 370 Calories, 16g fat, 55mg cholesterol, 250mg sodium, 33g carbohydrate, 7g fiber, 28g protein

Exchanges: 2 Carbohydrate, 4 Protein, 3 Fat

Grilled Bourbon Shrimp

Makes 4 servings.

4 wooden skewers

3 tablespoons pure maple syrup

3 tablespoons bourbon

1 tablespoon low-sodium soy sauce

1 tablespoon Dijon mustard

24 extra-large shrimp, peeled and deveined, tails on

½ red onion, cut into 1-inch pieces

24 1-inch pieces of fresh pineapple

¼ teaspoon Cajun seasoning

Seafood

1. Soak wooden skewers in water for 30 minutes. Preheat grill to medium heat.

2. Prepare sauce by combining maple syrup, bourbon, soy sauce, and Dijon mustard in medium bowl. Stir in shrimp and toss well. Allow to marinate for about 10 minutes.

3. Remove shrimp from marinade and thread on skewers, alternating with pieces of onion and pineapple. Season with Cajun seasoning. Grill over medium heat for 3 minutes on each side or until shrimp are cooked through.

4. Serve over brown rice seasoned with Cajun seasoning.

Nutrition Information: 200 calories, 0g fat, 215mg cholesterol, 350mg sodium, 17g carbohydrate, 1g fiber, 28g protein

Exchanges: 1 Carbohydrate, 4 Protein, 0 Fat

Cajun Tilapia with Lemon Dill Sauce

Makes 4 servings.

4 (approximately 5 oz. each) tilapia filets

¼ teaspoon fresh ground black pepper

1 tablespoon Cajun seasoning

1 tablespoon olive oil

1 lemon, thinly sliced

2 tablespoons light mayonnaise

¼ cup light sour cream

⅛ teaspoon garlic powder

1 teaspoon fresh lemon juice

1 tablespoon chopped fresh dill

1. Preheat oven to 350 degrees. Season filets with pepper and Cajun seasoning on both sides; set aside.

2. In large oven-proof skillet, heat olive oil. Add tilapia and cook over medium heat for 2 to 3 minutes to brown on each side. Remove from heat and place a layer of lemon slices over the fish filets.

3. Bake, uncovered, for 5 minutes or until fish flakes easily with a fork.

4. While the fish is baking, mix together mayonnaise, sour cream, garlic powder, lemon juice, and dill in a small bowl. Serve with tilapia.

Nutrition Information: 230 calories, 10g fat, 75mg cholesterol, 530mg sodium, 3g carbohydrate, 0g fiber, 30g protein

Exchanges: 0.5 Carbohydrate, 4.5 Protein, 2 Fat

Ginger Lime Red Snapper

Makes 4 servings.

2 cloves garlic, minced

½ teaspoon sriracha sauce

1 tablespoon grated fresh ginger

2 tablespoons fresh lime juice

2 tablespoons brown sugar

2 tablespoons fresh cilantro, chopped

1 ½ pounds red snapper filets

1 tablespoon sesame oil

2 tablespoons low-sodium soy sauce

1 lime, cut into wedges

1. Prepare charcoal grill. Lightly rub grill grate with oil to prevent sticking.

2. In mini food processor or blender, combine garlic, sriracha sauce, ginger, lime juice, brown sugar, and cilantro. Add 2 tablespoons of water and process until smooth. Pour ginger mixture into small bowl; set aside.

3. Combine sesame oil, soy sauce, and 1 tablespoon ginger mixture in shallow baking dish. Add fish filets, turning to coat. Cover with plastic wrap and refrigerate for 15 to 20 minutes.

4. Grill filets over medium-high heat for 4-5 minutes per side or until fish flakes easily with fork.

5. Serve with a squeeze of lime and drizzle evenly with remaining ginger-lime sauce.

Nutrition Information: 230 calories, 6g fat, 65mg cholesterol, 400mg sodium, 7g carbohydrate, 0g fiber, 36g protein

Exchanges: 0.5 Carbohydrate, 5 Protein, 1 Fat

Seafood

Lemon Dill Salmon

Makes 4 servings.

4 (approximately 5 oz. each) salmon filets

½ teaspoon salt

½ teaspoon fresh ground pepper

1 teaspoon chopped fresh dill or ½ teaspoon dill weed

1 lemon, sliced crosswise into 8 thin slices

Sauce:

3 tablespoons light sour cream

1 tablespoon light mayonnaise

½ teaspoon horseradish

½ teaspoon fresh lemon juice

½ teaspoon fresh lemon zest

½-1 teaspoon fresh (or dried) dill

1. Preheat oven to 425 degrees.

2. Place wire rack on foil-lined baking sheet. Place salmon filets skin side down onto rack. Sprinkle evenly with salt, pepper, and dill. Arrange 2 lemon slices on top of each filet.

3. Bake for 10 minutes or to desired degree of doneness—average rule of thumb for salmon is 10 minutes per 1-inch thickness, so time in oven will depend on thickness of salmon filets.

4. While salmon is baking, in small bowl, stir together sour cream, mayonnaise, horseradish, lemon juice, zest, and dill.

5. Remove salmon from oven and serve with dollop of lemon dill sauce.

Nutrition Information: 260 calories, 13g fat, 95mg cholesterol, 400mg sodium, 1g carbohydrate, 0g fiber, 32g protein

Exchanges: 1 Carbohydrate, 4.5 Protein, 2.5 Fat

Dill weed is rich in flavonoid antioxidants and has been shown to have antibacterial properties. Combine dill with your favorite plain yogurt, chopped cucumber, red wine vinegar, and garlic for a speedy and nutritious veggie dip!

Green Tea Shrimp with Lemon Ginger Sauce

Makes 4 servings.

28 extra-large shrimp

1 cup water

2 ginger-flavored green tea bags

1 teaspoon lemon zest

¼ cup fresh lemon juice

2 tablespoons honey

2 teaspoons grated fresh ginger

1 tablespoon low-sodium tamari sauce

2 cloves garlic, minced

1 tablespoon olive oil

½ teaspoon lemon pepper blend

2 tablespoons chopped fresh cilantro

2 cups cooked brown rice

1. Peel and devein shrimp, leaving tails on.

2. Bring water to boil; add tea bags and let steep for 2 to 3 minutes.

3. In medium bowl, combine cooled tea, lemon zest, lemon juice, honey, ginger, tamari sauce, and garlic; set aside.

4. Heat oil over medium-high heat in large sauté pan. Add shrimp and sprinkle with lemon pepper. Sear on one side; turn shrimp and add tea sauce to pan. Simmer for 2 minutes; add cilantro and continue to simmer over low heat for additional minute.

5. Remove shrimp and cook sauce over medium heat until reduced by about half. Place shrimp back in sauce. Serve over brown rice.

Nutrition Information: 280 calories, 5g fat, 170mg cholesterol, 380mg sodium, 39g carbohydrate, 2g fiber, 21g protein

Exchanges: 2.5 carbohydrate, 3 protein, 1 fat

Ginger is a spice used in cuisines around the world, and is well known for its ability to relax the gastrointestinal tract and treat an unsettled stomach. Ginger root contains potent anti-inflammatory compounds, gingerols, which are effective in alleviating pain and swelling related to arthritis.

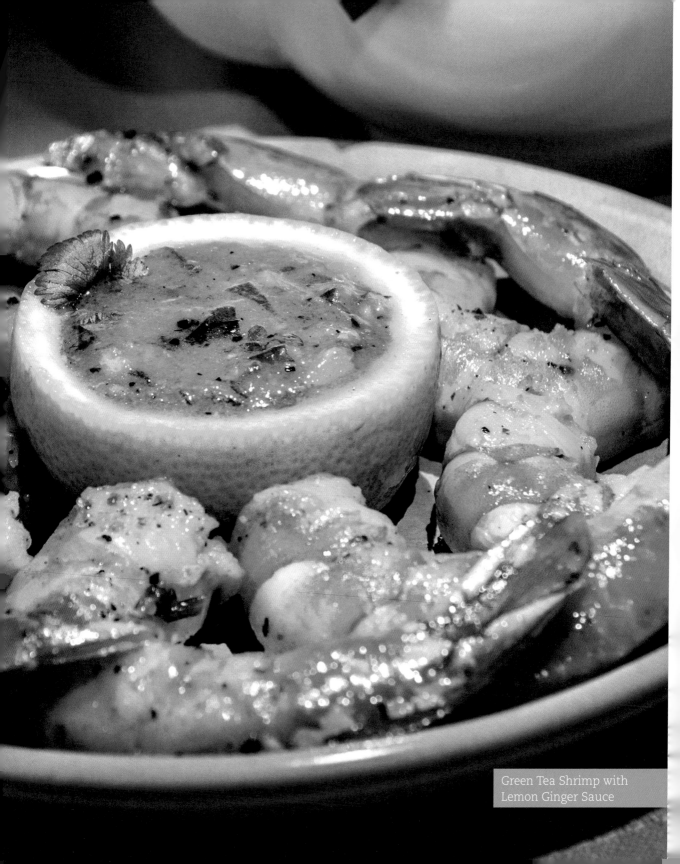

Green Tea Shrimp with
Lemon Ginger Sauce

Orange Basil Grilled Salmon

Makes 6 servings.

2 teaspoons grated orange rind

¼ cup fresh orange juice

2 tablespoons fresh lemon juice

2 tablespoons extra-virgin olive oil

⅓ cup chopped fresh basil

6 (approximately 5 oz. each) salmon filets

1. Combine orange rind, orange juice, lemon juice, olive oil, and basil in a large plastic zippered bag; add salmon. Seal and chill for 1 hour.

2. Remove salmon and discard marinade. Place salmon, skin side up, on grill rack over medium hot coals. Cover with grill lid and cook about 7-8 minutes; turn and continue cooking an additional 3-4 minutes with skin side down to desired degree of doneness. Carefully remove salmon from grill, leaving skin on grill, and serve.

Nutrition Information: 230 calories, 10g fat, 90mg cholesterol, 70mg sodium, 0g carbohydrate, 0g fiber, 32g protein

Exchanges: 0 Carbohydrates, 4.5 Protein, 2 Fat

Citrus juice and zest are powerful anti-inflammatories, and when combined with salmon and herbs they act to significantly boost the absorption of the many anti-inflammatory benefits in this dish!

Seafood

Parmesan Crusted Red Snapper

Makes 4 servings.

½ cup panko bread crumbs

2 tablespoons grated Parmesan cheese

1 teaspoon lemon-pepper seasoning

¼ teaspoon salt

4 (approximately 5 oz. each) red snapper filets

2 tablespoons olive oil

Jalapeño Tartar Sauce:

⅓ cup low-fat mayonnaise

2 teaspoons fresh lime juice

1 tablespoon finely chopped pickled jalapeño pepper

¼ teaspoon lime zest

¼ teaspoon ground cumin

⅛ teaspoon salt

1. To prepare sauce, combine mayonnaise, lime juice, jalapeño, lime zest, cumin, and salt in small bowl. Stir until well blended. Cover and chill until ready to serve.

2. In a shallow bowl, combine the bread crumbs, cheese, lemon-pepper, and salt; add filets, one at a time, and turn to coat.

3. Heat oil in a heavy skillet over medium heat; sauté filets in batches for 4-5 minutes on each side or until fish flakes easily with a fork. Serve with Jalapeño Tartar Sauce.

Nutrition Information: 280 calories, 16g fat, 50mg cholesterol, 520mg sodium, 8g carbohydrate, 0g fiber, 26g protein

Exchanges: 0.5 Carbohydrate, 3.5 Protein, 3 Fat

Pecan Crusted Honey Dijon Salmon

Makes 4 servings.

4 (approximately 4 oz. each) salmon filets

1 tablespoon honey

1 tablespoon coarse-grain Dijon mustard

1 tablespoon olive oil

¼ teaspoon salt

¼ teaspoon each salt and fresh cracked black pepper

⅓ cup whole wheat panko bread crumbs

¼ cup chopped pecans

2 tablespoons chopped fresh parsley

Seafood

1. Preheat oven to 450 degrees.

2. Pat salmon with paper towels. Place skin side down in a shallow baking dish coated with cooking spray.

3. Combine honey, mustard, olive oil, salt, and pepper in a small bowl. Brush mustard mixture over top of salmon.

4. In small bowl, combine bread crumbs, pecans, and parsley. Sprinkle pecan mixture over top of salmon.

5. Bake salmon for approximately 10 minutes per inch or desired degree of doneness.

Nutrition Information: 310 calories, 17g fat, 70mg cholesterol, 300mg sodium, 11g carbohydrate, 1g fiber, 27g protein

Exchanges: 1 Carbohydrate, 4 Protein, 3 Fat

Believe it! Honey is more than a delicious natural sweetener. It is also a source of antioxidants and a proven treatment for sore throats. Remember, it is a source of added sugar, so use sparingly!

Pecan Crusted Halibut

Makes 4 servings.

¼ cup all-purpose flour

½ teaspoon each salt and fresh ground black pepper

2 teaspoons coarse-grain Dijon mustard

1 large egg

¼ cup pecans, chopped

¾ cup whole wheat panko bread crumbs

4 (approximately 4 oz. each) skinless halibut filets

2 tablespoons olive oil

Optional: Dijon Cream Sauce

1. Combine flour, salt, and pepper in a shallow bowl. Whisk mustard and egg in another shallow bowl. Combine pecans and bread crumbs in a third shallow bowl.

2. Dredge each halibut filet in flour mixture, shaking off excess. Dip halibut in egg mixture to coat; drain excess. Place halibut in pecan mixture, pressing slightly to coat both sides of the filet.

3. In large nonstick skillet, heat olive oil over medium heat. Add filets, in batches, and cook 2 minutes on each side or until lightly browned. Arrange filets on a foil-lined baking sheet. Bake at 350 degrees for 10 minutes or until done.

4. Remove halibut from oven, drizzle with sauce if desired, and serve immediately.

Nutrition Information: 240 calories, 12g fat, 75mg cholesterol, 250mg sodium, 9g carbohydrate, 1g fiber, 24g protein

Exchanges: 0.5 Carbohydrate, 3.5 Protein, 2.5 Fat

Dijon Cream Sauce

¼ cup half and half

2 tablespoons coarse grain Dijon mustard

⅛ teaspoon each salt and fresh ground black pepper

While halibut is finishing in oven, prepare sauce by placing half and half, Dijon mustard, salt, and pepper in small saucepan. Place over low heat, whisking constantly until heated through.

Nutrition Information: 30 calories, 3g fat, 5mg cholesterol, 230mg sodium, 2g carbohydrate, 0g fiber, 1g protein

Exchanges: 0 Carbohydrate, 0 Protein, 1 Fat

Hot 'n' Crunchy Trout

Makes 4 servings.

4 (approximately 5 oz. each) trout filets

½ teaspoon each salt and fresh ground black pepper

2 tablespoons flour

¾ cup whole wheat panko bread crumbs

¼ cup chopped toasted pecans

1 tablespoon crushed red pepper flakes

1 egg

½ cup milk

2 tablespoons olive oil

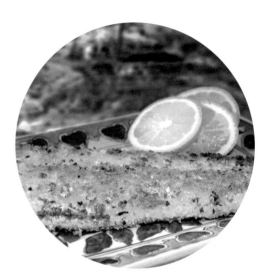

Hot 'n' Crunchy Trout

1. Preheat oven to 425 degrees.

2. Season trout filets with salt and pepper, dredge lightly in flour shaking off excess; set aside.

3. In shallow dish, combine breadcrumbs, pecans, and red pepper flakes; set aside.

4. In separate shallow dish, whisk together egg and milk. Dip trout in egg wash then into crumb mixture, pressing crumbs firmly into flesh-side of trout.

5. In heavy, oven-proof skillet, heat olive oil over medium heat. Place trout, flesh side down, in hot skillet. Brown for 2-3 minutes. Turn carefully and put skillet into oven for 3 to 4 minutes or until fish flakes easily with fork.

Nutrition Information: 330 calories, 18g fat, 110mg cholesterol, 400mg sodium, 10g carbohydrate, 2g fiber, 33g protein

Exchanges: 0.5 carbohydrate, 4.5 protein, 3.5 fat

Pistachio Coconut Crusted Salmon

Makes 4 servings.

4 (approximately 4 oz. each) skinless salmon filets

2 teaspoons orange-lemon pepper blend

2 tablespoons chopped pistachios

2 tablespoons unsweetened coconut

⅓ cup whole wheat panko breadcrumbs

1. Preheat oven to 425 degrees. Grind pepper blend evenly over both sides of salmon filets; set aside.

2. In small bowl, combine chopped pistachios, coconut, and breadcrumbs.

3. Place salmon on baking sheet and sprinkle evenly with bread crumb mixture. Bake for approximately 10 minutes per inch or to desired degree of doneness.

Nutrition Information: 230 calories, 11g fat, 70mg cholesterol, 125mg sodium, 6g carbohydrate, 1 g fiber, 27g protein

Exchanges: 0.5 Carbohydrate, 4 Protein, 2 Fat

Red Snapper Veracruz

Makes 4 servings

4 (approximately 5 oz. each) red snapper filets, cut into 4 pieces

½ teaspoon salt

1 lime

1 tablespoon olive oil

1 white onion, chopped

3 garlic cloves, chopped

1 (28 oz.) can whole tomatoes, drained

10 large green manzanilla olives, pitted and chopped

2 tablespoons capers

2 pickled jalapeño peppers, chopped

2 tablespoons pickled jalapeño juice

2 tablespoons fresh parsley, chopped

2 sprigs fresh marjoram, optional

½ teaspoon dried Mexican oregano

2 bay leaves

Freshly ground black pepper

Optional: Corn tortillas, warmed

1. Sprinkle filets with salt and place in a shallow pan. Cut lime in half and squeeze over filets. Place lime halves in pan, cover, and marinate in refrigerator for 1 hour.

2. Heat oil in a large sauté pan over medium-low heat. Add onions and cook until transparent, about 10 minutes. Stir in garlic and cook for 1 minute.

3. Coarsely chop tomatoes and add to onion mixture; cook for 5 minutes. Add olives, capers, jalapeño peppers, jalapeño juice, parsley, marjoram, oregano, and bay leaves. Season with pepper; cook over low heat for 20 minutes.

4. Add filets, lime juice, and limes to tomato mixture. Cover and cook, turning once, for 4-5 minutes per side.

Discard bay leaves and limes. Serve immediately with tortillas, if desired.

Nutrition Information: 250 calories, 6g fat, 50mg cholesterol, 930mg sodium, 16g carbohydrate, 4g fiber, 32g protein

Exchanges: 1 Carbohydrate, 4.5 Protein, 1 Fat

Tuscan Shrimp with Lemon Orzo

Makes 6 servings.

Tuscan Shrimp:

¼ cup olive oil

¼ cup fresh lemon juice

1 teaspoon each salt and fresh
  ground pepper

1 teaspoon dry mustard

2 teaspoons Dijon mustard

2 cloves garlic, lightly crushed

1 small onion, diced

½ cup Tuscan Pepperoncini, chopped

½ cup fresh basil, minced

1 ½ pounds extra-large shrimp (approximately 20 shrimp), peeled and deveined

4 skewers

Lemon Orzo:

8 ounces whole wheat orzo pasta

1 tablespoon olive oil

Zest of 1 lemon

Juice of 1 lemon

2 tablespoons freshly grated Parmigia-
  no-Reggiano cheese

¼ teaspoon each salt and fresh
  ground pepper

1. Whisk together the olive oil, lemon juice, salt, pepper, and mustards in a medium bowl. Stir in the garlic, onions, Pepperocini, and basil. Add the shrimp and toss to coat. Cover and refrigerate for 1 hour.

2. Cook and drain the orzo according to package instructions. Place the orzo in a bowl, add the olive oil, and let cool to room temperature. Add the lemon zest and juice to the orzo. Stir in the cheese and season with salt and pepper.

3. Preheat the grill to medium-high. Remove the shrimp from the marinade and thread onto the skewers, through the head and tail. Discard the marinade. Grill for 2 to 3 minutes per side or until the shrimp turn pink. Serve over the Lemon Orzo.

Nutrition Information: 270 calories, 6g fat, 170mg cholesterol, 380mg sodium, 29g carbohydrate, 2g fiber, 24g protein

Exchanges: 2 Carbohydrate, 3.5 Protein, 1 Fat

When life gives you lemons, make marinade! Lemons are a rich source of Vitamin C, and antioxidant and anti-inflammatory properties, and are uniquely recognized for being able to boost the absorption of AI when added to any recipe.

Roasted Salmon with Avocado Grapefruit Salsa

Makes 4 servings.

4 (approximately 4 oz. each) salmon filets

1 teaspoon olive oil

½ teaspoon each salt and fresh ground black pepper

1 teaspoon ancho chile powder

1 large grapefruit

1 small avocado, pitted, peeled, and cubed

1 jalapeño, seeded and minced

2 tablespoons red onion, minced

2 tablespoons cilantro, minced

1 tablespoon fresh lime juice

1. Preheat oven to 400 degrees. In glass baking dish, place the salmon skin side down. Brush top with olive oil. Sprinkle with salt, pepper, and ancho chile powder. Place in oven and roast until almost opaque in the center, about 10-12 minutes.

2. While salmon cooks, peel and section grapefruit over small bowl. (Use a sharp knife to cut between the membranes to release grapefruit segments into the bowl.)

3. Cut grapefruit segments crosswise into ½-inch pieces; return to the bowl.

4. Gently mix in the avocado, jalapeño, onion, cilantro, and lime juice.

5. Gently lift salmon off skin and place salmon filets on serving plate. Spoon the grapefruit mixture over salmon and serve.

Nutrition Information: 310 calories, 16g fat, 70mg cholesterol, 360mg sodium, 14g carbohydrate, 5g fiber, 28g protein

Exchanges: 1 carbohydrate, 4 protein, 3 fat

Grapefruit has significant anti-inflammatory health benefits related to its ability to reduce cholesterol and triglyceride levels.

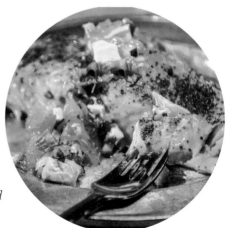

Roasted Salmon with Avocado Grapefruit Salsa

Sesame-Crusted Tuna with Wasabi Vinaigrette

Makes 4 servings.

2 tablespoons low-sodium tamari sauce

1 ½ tablespoons canola oil

2 (approximately 8 oz. each) ahi tuna steaks

1 tablespoon each of black and white sesame seeds

½ teaspoon ground coriander

¼ teaspoon sea salt

Wasabi Vinaigrette:

1 teaspoon wasabi paste

1 ½ tablespoons rice wine vinegar

1 tablespoon sesame oil

1 tablespoon low-sodium soy sauce

1 tablespoon mirin

2 teaspoons fresh ginger, grated

Salad:

6 cups salad greens

1 small avocado, sliced

1 cup cucumber, sliced

½ cup carrot, julienned

½ cup edamame

2 green onions, sliced

2 tablespoons pickled ginger

1. Blend tamari sauce with ½ tablespoon of oil. Place tuna steaks in tamari mixture and turn to coat; set aside to marinate.

2. In small bowl, combine sesame seeds and seasonings; press evenly over both sides of tuna steaks.

3. Heat 1 tablespoon of oil in a 12-inch nonstick skillet over medium heat. Cook tuna 2-3 minutes per side. Use care not to overcook tuna; it is best eaten rare. The center should still have a dark pink color. Remove steaks from heat and let sit for 2 to 3 minutes before slicing into thin slices.

4. In small bowl, combine ingredients for Wasabi Vinaigrette; set aside.

5. Arrange ingredients for salad on 4 serving plates. Top with tuna slices and drizzle with vinaigrette just before serving.

Nutrition Information: 330 calories, 17g fat, 45mg cholesterol, 790mg sodium, 17g carbohydrate, 7g fiber, 30g protein

Exchanges: 1 carbohydrate, 4.5 protein, 3.5 fat

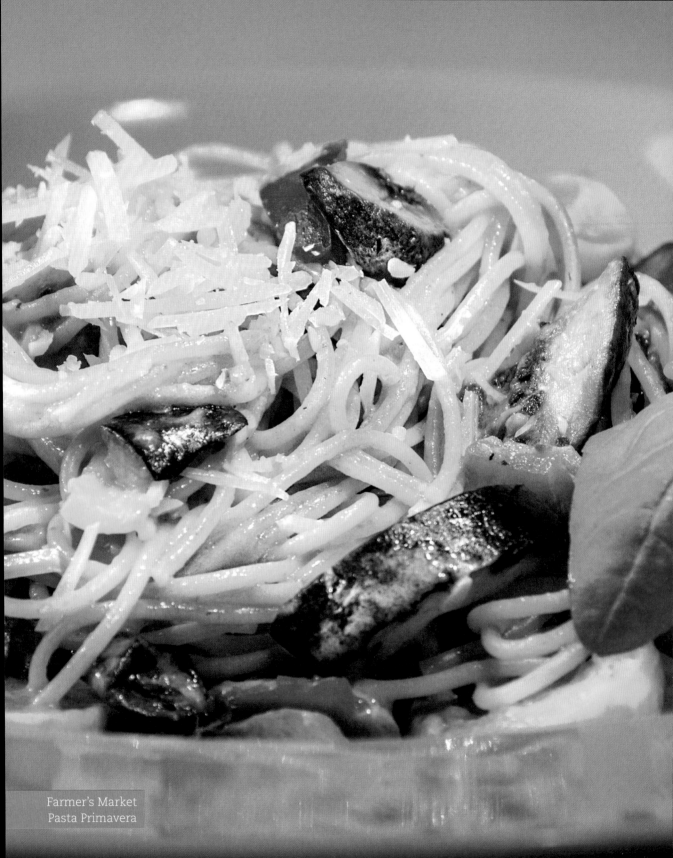

Farmer's Market
Pasta Primavera

Farmer's Market Pasta Primavera

Makes 4 servings.

Ingredients:

6 cups of your favorite assorted vegetables, cut into 1-inch pieces (*I used zucchini, yellow squash, red onion, multi-colored bell peppers, baby bella mushrooms, spinach, and heirloom tomatoes.*)

1 tablespoon olive oil

2 cloves garlic, minced

¼ cup fresh basil, cut into strips

Juice from 1 fresh lemon

½ cup dry white wine

½ teaspoon fresh ground black pepper

6 ounces angel hair pasta (*I used fresh lemon pepper pasta from the Farmer's Market.*)

2 tablespoons olive oil

¼ cup fresh grated Parmesan cheese

Optional: 2 cups cooked chicken, diced*

Directions:

1. Prepare your choice of vegetables by cutting into approximately 1-inch pieces.

2. In large skillet, heat olive oil over high heat. Add vegetables and garlic and cook, stirring constantly, until crisp tender. Stir in basil, lemon juice, wine, and pepper; simmer for 3 minutes.

3. While vegetables are cooking, bring water to boil in large pot. Add pasta and cook to al dente. Drain well and add pasta to vegetable mixture.

4. Toss with olive oil and cheese and serve immediately.

*Adding 2 cups of cooked chicken will give you an additional 20 grams of protein for a total of 4.5 protein servings.

Nutrition Information: 320 calories, 10g fat, 20mg cholesterol, 160mg sodium, 42g carbohydrate, 4g fiber, 13g protein

Exchanges: 3 Carbohydrate, 2 Protein, 2 Fat

7-Layer Mediterranean Dip

Makes 12 servings.

1 (10 oz.) container roasted red pepper hummus

2 cups chopped spinach/romaine lettuce blend

¾ cup chopped tomatoes

¾ cup chopped, peeled, and seeded cucumbers

¼ cup finely chopped red onions

½ cup crumbled reduced-fat feta cheese

3 tablespoons chopped Kalamata olives

Optional: fresh-cut veggies, whole grain crackers, or pita triangles

1. Spread hummus on serving platter. Layer spinach blend, tomatoes, cucumbers, red onions, cheese, and olives on top of hummus.

2. Serve with fresh veggies, whole grain crackers, or pita triangles, if desired.

Nutrition Information: 60 calories, 3.5g fat, 0mg cholesterol, 220mg sodium, 6g carbohydrate, 1g fiber, 2g protein

Exchanges: 0.5 Carbohydrate, 0.5 Protein, 0.5 Fat

Olives are rich in anti-inflammatory fatty acids. Toss a handful into your favorite pasta dishes, onto a salad, or just enjoy plain.

Parmesan Risotto with Mushrooms & Spinach

Makes 4 servings.

4 cups low-sodium vegetable broth

2 tablespoons olive oil, divided

1 cup Arborio rice

½ cup white wine

2 teaspoons minced garlic

1 cup sliced fresh mushrooms

¼ cup chopped green onion

½ teaspoon crushed red chile pepper flakes

1 (14 oz.) bag fresh baby spinach

½ cup freshly grated Parmesan cheese

½ teaspoon fresh ground black pepper

1. In medium saucepan, bring broth to a boil.

2. While broth comes to a boil, heat 1 tablespoon of olive oil in a large heavy-bottomed saucepan over medium-high heat. Pour in the rice, and stir until the rice is coated in oil and has started to toast, 2 to 3 minutes. Reduce heat to medium; add wine, stir, and simmer until absorbed.

3. Stir in one-third of the boiling vegetable broth; continue stirring until incorporated. Repeat this process twice more, stirring constantly. Incorporating the broth should take 15 to 20 minutes.

4. While you are cooking the rice, heat the remaining tablespoon of oil in a pan. Stir in garlic, mushrooms, green onion, and red chili flakes and cook for 5 minutes. Add spinach and cook an additional 5 minutes. Add Parmesan cheese and season with black pepper.

5. Divide risotto evenly into four bowls. Top with vegetable mixture and serve.

Nutrition Information: 370 calories, 12g fat, 15mg cholesterol, 770mg sodium, 47g carbohydrate, 6g fiber, 13g protein

Exchanges: 3 Carbohydrate, 2 Protein, 2 Fat

Spinach is a potent source of antioxidants. Try switching romaine lettuce for spinach in salads and sandwiches for an extra burst of color, vitamin K, Vitamin C, and iron.

Pepper Jack Quinoa Risotto

Makes 8 servings.

7 cups low-sodium vegetable broth

1 tablespoon extra-virgin olive oil

½ cup shallot, diced

2 cloves garlic, minced

1 bay leaf

1 teaspoon each ground cumin and ground coriander

2 cups quinoa, washed

½ cup green onions, thinly sliced

4 ounces pepper jack cheese, shredded

½ teaspoon hot pepper sauce

2 cups fresh roasted corn (frozen can be used)

¾ cup roasted red bell peppers (fresh or from jar), chopped

1 tablespoon lemon juice

½ teaspoon each salt and fresh ground black pepper

1. Pour broth into saucepan and bring just to a simmer; hold at this temperature.

2. Heat oil in large saucepan over medium-high heat. Add shallots and garlic and sweat about 2 min. Do not let them brown. Add bay leaf, spices, and quinoa. Toast lightly, stirring constantly. When you feel each kernel is coated in oil and spices are very fragrant, begin adding stock. Stir in 1-2 ladles of stock at a time. Stir constantly. Do not add more broth until the last amount has cooked out. This should take about 20 minutes.

3. Stir in green onions, cheese, hot sauce, corn, bell peppers, lemon juice, salt, and pepper. Cook an additional 3 minutes or until hot throughout. Remove bay leaf and serve.

Nutrition Information: 310 calories, 9g fat, 15mg cholesterol, 380mg sodium, 47g carbohydrate, 6g fiber, 12g protein

Exchanges: 3 Carbohydrate, 2 Protein, 2 Fat

Quinoa is much higher in protein and dietary fiber than brown rice. Try switching brown rice for quinoa in some of your favorite recipes!

Stuffed Poblano Peppers

Makes 8 servings.

1 (28 oz.) can crushed tomatoes

1-2 cloves garlic, minced

1 chipotle pepper packed in adobo sauce, minced

1 tablespoon olive oil

½ cup diced onion

½ cup diced red bell pepper

1 (15 oz.) can pinto beans, drained and rinsed

1 (8.5 oz.) package microwavable quinoa/ brown rice blend

1 teaspoon chili powder

4 medium poblano peppers

1 cup reduced-fat pepper jack cheese shreds

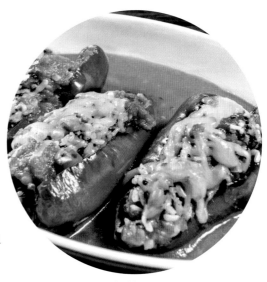

Stuffed Poblano Peppers

1. Place tomatoes, garlic, and chipotle pepper in saucepan and simmer over low heat for about 10 minutes; set aside.

2. In large skillet, heat olive oil over medium-high heat. Add onion and bell pepper; sauté about 5 minutes. Stir in beans, quinoa, and chili powder.

3. Split poblano peppers in half and remove seeds. Stuff the peppers with quinoa mixture.

4. Ladle half of crushed tomato mixture into 9 × 13-inch glass baking dish. Place peppers on top and ladle with the remaining sauce. Cover and bake at 400 degrees for 30 minutes. Remove cover, sprinkle with cheese, and bake an additional 5 minutes.

Nutrition Information: 280 calories, 7g fat, 10mg cholesterol, 440mg sodium, 43g carbohydrate, 4g fiber, 13g protein

Exchanges: 3 Carbohydrate, 2 Protein, 1 Fat

Skillet Gnocchi with Chard & White Beans

Makes 8 servings.

1 tablespoon extra-virgin olive oil

1 (16 oz.) package whole wheat gnocchi

1 teaspoon extra-virgin olive oil

1 small onion, thinly sliced

2 garlic cloves, minced

½ cup water

6 cups Swiss chard or spinach leaves, chopped

1 (15 oz.) can diced tomatoes with Italian seasoning

1 (15 oz.) can cannellini beans, drained and rinsed

½ teaspoon fresh ground black pepper

1 cup part-skim mozzarella cheese, shredded

¼ cup Parmesan cheese, shredded

1. Heat 1 tablespoon olive oil in large skillet over medium heat. Add gnocchi and cook, stirring often until plumped and starting to brown, 5-7 minutes. Transfer to bowl.

2. To same skillet, add remaining 1 teaspoon olive oil, onion, and garlic; cook, stirring often, over medium heat for 2 minutes. Return gnocchi to skillet. Add water, cover, and cook until onion is soft for about 5 minutes. Add chard or spinach and continue stirring until starting to wilt. Stir in tomatoes, beans, and pepper; bring to a simmer.

3. Sprinkle with cheeses, cover, and cook until cheese is melted.

Nutrition information: 350 calories, 9g fat, 20mg cholesterol, 770mg sodium, 50g carbohydrate, 6g fiber, 16g protein

Exchanges: 3.5 Carbohydrate, 2.5 Protein, 2 Fat

Beans are a high-fiber way to add color, texture, and protein to pastas, salads, and side dishes.

Skillet Mexican Quinoa

Makes 8 servings.

1 tablespoon olive oil

2 cloves garlic, minced

1 jalapeño, minced

1 (8.8 oz.) package microwavable red and white quinoa

1 (15 oz.) can black beans, drained and rinsed

1 (14.5 oz.) can diced tomatoes with green chilies

1 cup corn kernels, fresh or frozen

1 teaspoon each chili powder and cumin

Juice of 1 lime

½ teaspoon each salt and fresh ground black pepper

1 small avocado, peeled and cubed

2 tablespoons chopped fresh cilantro leaves

1. Heat olive oil in large skillet over medium heat.

2. Add garlic and jalapeño to pan and stir frequently until fragrant (about 1 minute).

3. Microwave quinoa according to package directions. Stir in quinoa, beans, tomatoes, corn, chili powder, and cumin.

4. Bring to a simmer; cover, reduce heat, and cook over low heat about 5 minutes.

5. Stir in lime juice, salt, and pepper.

6. Garnish with avocado and cilantro.

Nutrition Information: 180 calories, 6g fat, 0mg cholesterol, 400mg sodium, 25g carbohydrate, 8g fiber, 6g protein

Exchanges: 2 Carbohydrate, 1 Protein, 1 Fat

Garlic is an herb best known for adding flavor to food. However, its anti-inflammatory properties make it a useful treatment for a variety of conditions from high blood pressure to arthritis!

Vegetarian Creole Gumbo

Makes 6 servings.

3 tablespoons canola oil

3 tablespoons flour

2 cups chopped onion

1 teaspoon salt

¼ cup sliced green onions

3 cloves garlic, minced

3 dried bay leaves

¼ teaspoon cayenne pepper

1 cup diced celery

½ cup sliced carrots

5 cups organic vegetable stock

1 (10 oz.) bag frozen black-eyed peas

1 ½ cups cooked brown rice

1 cup frozen cut okra

2 cups chopped fresh mixed spinach and kale

¼ cup chopped fresh parsley

1. In large Dutch oven, heat oil over medium-high heat. Add flour and whisk to make a smooth paste. Cook, stirring constantly, for about 5 minutes; then reduce heat and cook another 3-5 minutes, stirring until roux is golden brown.

2. Add onions and salt and cook on medium heat for 5 minutes, stirring frequently. Add green onion, garlic, bay leaves, cayenne, celery, and carrots. Add vegetable stock and bring to a boil.

3. Add black-eyed peas, rice, and okra. Cover and reduce heat to simmer for 20 minutes. Remove lid and stir in spinach/kale mixture and parsley; simmer for 5 minutes.

4. Remove bay leaves, adjust seasonings as needed, and serve.

Nutrition Information: 260 calories, 8g fat, 0mg cholesterol, 920mg sodium, 41g carbohydrate, 7g fiber, 8g protein

Exchanges: 2.5 Carbohydrate, 1 Protein, 1.5 Fat

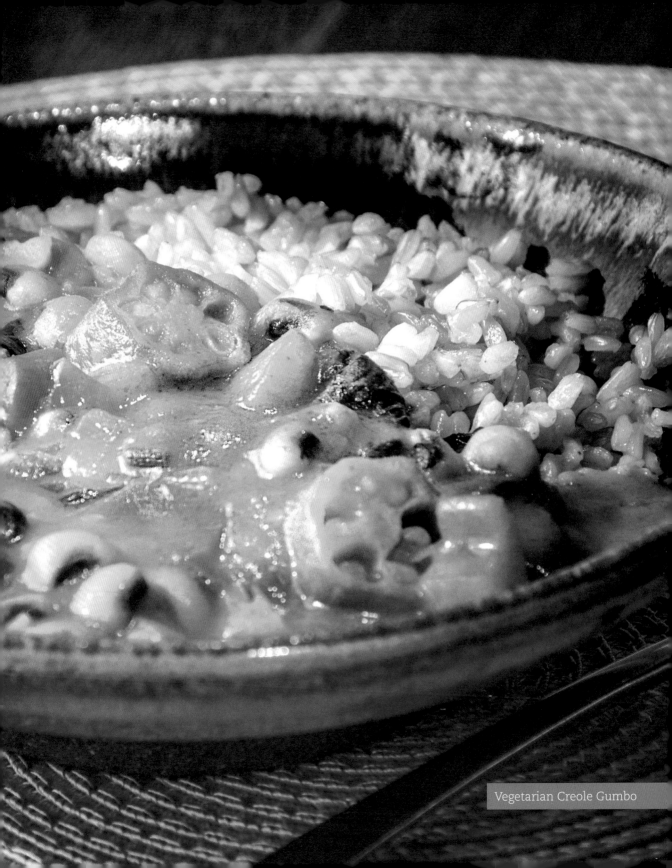

Vegetarian Creole Gumbo

Spinach Artichoke Pasta

Makes 4 servings.

2 tablespoons olive oil, divided

2 cloves garlic, minced

1 (10 oz.) bag baby spinach

1 (15 oz.) can artichoke hearts, drained
  and cut in half

1 tablespoon flour

1 ½ cups 1% milk

¼ cup grated Parmesan cheese

1 cup mozzarella cheese, shredded

¼ teaspoon cayenne pepper and salt

½ teaspoon fresh ground black pepper

2 cups whole wheat penne pasta,
  cooked to al dente

Crushed red pepper to taste

¼ cup seasoned panko bread crumbs

1. In large skillet, heat 1 tablespoon olive oil over medium heat. Add garlic and spinach. Cook and stir until wilted; about one minute. Place spinach in large bowl and set aside.

2. In same skillet, add remaining 1 tablespoon olive oil and place over high heat. Add artichokes, cook, and stir for about 2 minutes. Place artichokes in bowl with spinach.

3. Reduce heat to low; add flour to pan drippings, whisking until smooth. Pour in milk, whisk to combine, and let cook for 3 minutes or until mixture begins to thicken. Add cheeses, cayenne pepper, salt, and black pepper and stir to melt.

4. Stir spinach, artichokes, and pasta into sauce, tossing gently to combine. Place in serving bowl, top with crushed red pepper and bread crumbs to serve.

Nutrition Information: 380 calories, 16g fat, 25mg cholesterol, 650mg sodium, 41g carbohydrate, 11g fiber, 21g protein

Exchanges: 3 Carbohydrate, 3 Protein, 3 Fat

Vegetarian Bolognese

Makes 6 servings.

1 tablespoon olive oil

1 cup chopped onion

½ teaspoon each fresh ground black pepper and salt

4 cups eggplant (cut into 1-inch cubes)

3 carrots, sliced thin

1 medium zucchini, cut into 1/4-inch slices

2 cloves minced garlic

2 cups whole grain penne pasta

1 tablespoon tomato paste

½ cup red wine

1 (28 oz.) can crushed tomatoes

¼ cup mascarpone cheese

1 teaspoon chopped fresh oregano (or ½ teaspoon dried)

2 tablespoons chopped fresh basil

¼ cup Parmesan cheese

Optional: ¼ teaspoon crushed red pepper flakes

1. In large Dutch oven, heat olive oil over medium high heat. Stir in onion, sprinkle with salt and pepper, and cook over low heat until transparent. Stir in eggplant, carrots, zucchini, and garlic. Stir and cook over low heat until vegetables are crisp tender.

2. While vegetables are cooking, bring large pot of salted water to boil for pasta. Cook to al dente; drain pasta, reserving 1 cup of pasta water to add to sauce.

3. Add tomato paste, red wine, crushed tomatoes, and 1 cup pasta water to vegetables in Dutch oven; stir until blended. Cook over low heat until liquid is reduced by about half, about 5-10 minutes.

4. Stir in mascarpone cheese, oregano, basil, and cooked pasta. Toss with Parmesan cheese and serve.

Nutrition Information: 330 calories, 14g fat, 25mg cholesterol, 570mg sodium, 44g carbohydrate, 9g fiber, 13g protein

Exchanges: 3 Carbohydrate, 2 Protein, 3 Fat

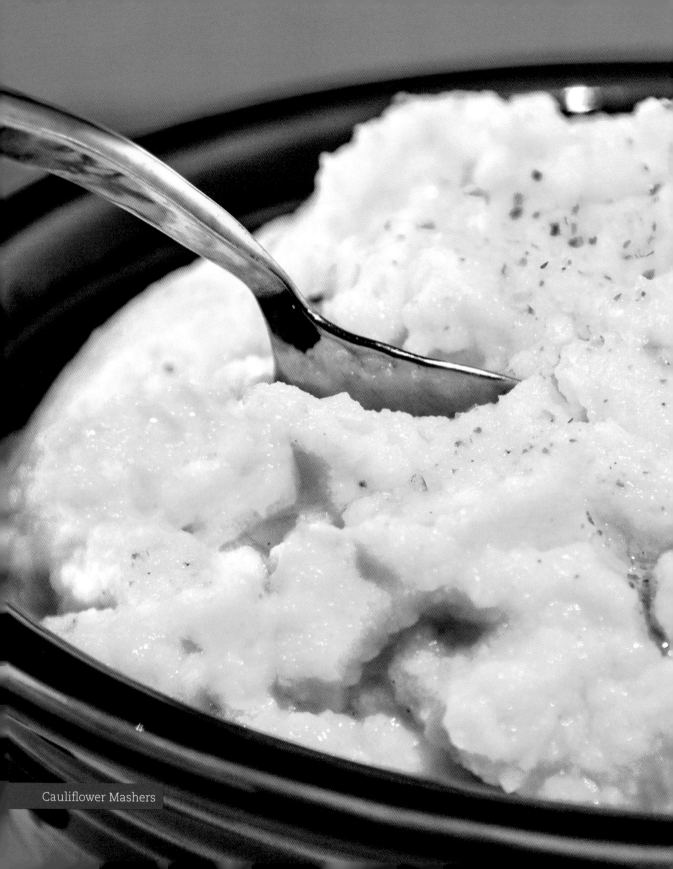

Cauliflower Mashers

Cauliflower Mashers

Makes 4 servings.

Ingredients:

1 head cauliflower

2 cups low-sodium chicken stock

3 cloves garlic

¼ cup Parmesan cheese

2 tablespoons half and half

½ teaspoon each salt and fresh ground black pepper

Directions:

1. Remove bottom and outer leaves of cauliflower; break cauliflower into florets.

2. Bring stock to a boil. Add cauliflower and garlic cloves. Boil for 7 minutes or until tender. Drain well; reserve ½ cup of liquid.

3. In a bowl with an immersion blender, or in a food processor, puree the cooked cauliflower, garlic, Parmesan, and half and half until smooth. Use reserved cooking stock to create desired consistency. Add salt and pepper; serve immediately.

Nutrition Information: 70 calories, 2.5g fat, 5mg cholesterol, 480mg sodium, 9g carbohydrate, 4g fiber, 5g protein

Exchanges: 0.5 Carbohydrate, 0.5 Protein, 0.5 Fat

Cauliflower revival: The lowly cauliflower is typically blanketed in cheese sauce and merely endured rather than enjoyed. At a mere 27 calories per cup, cauliflower is a rich source of vitamin C, vitamin K, folate, and fiber. This versatile veg deserves more recognition. Your family will love these mock mashed potatoes and you can feel great about serving them.

Oven Roasted Vegetables

Makes 4 servings.

2 cups broccoli florets

2 cups cauliflower florets

1 red bell pepper, cut into 1-inch pieces

2 cups cremini (baby bella) mushrooms, halved

1 small red onion, cut in half and quartered

2 medium yellow squash, quartered and cut into 1-inch pieces

3 cloves garlic, minced

2 tablespoons olive oil

2 tablespoons balsamic vinegar

½ teaspoon each sea salt and fresh cracked black pepper

1. Preheat oven to 425 degrees.

2. Spray large jelly roll pan with cooking spray. Place cut vegetables onto pan, drizzle with olive oil, toss gently, and place in oven.

3. Cook for 15 minutes, stopping to toss vegetables every 5 minutes during cooking time.

4. Remove from oven; drizzle with balsamic vinegar. Sprinkle with salt and pepper and serve.

Nutrition Information: 140 calories, 7g fat, 0mg cholesterol, 330mg sodium, 16g carbohydrate, 5g fiber, 5g protein

Exchanges: 1 Carbohydrate, 0.5 Protein, 1 Fat

A photo of these vegetables appears with Asian Flank Steak.

Crispy Parmesan Roasted Broccoli

Makes 4 servings.

- 1 ½ pounds fresh broccoli
- ½ teaspoon salt
- ½ cup grated Parmesan cheese
- 2 tablespoons fresh lemon juice

1. Preheat oven to 400 degrees.
2. Trim ends off broccoli and cut lengthwise into spears
3. Fill large pot with water and salt, and bring to a boil. Add broccoli to boiling water and blanch for about 3 minutes. Pour into colander to drain.
4. Pat broccoli dry with paper towels and place on jelly roll pan in single layer. Sprinkle cheese evenly over broccoli and place in oven for about 10 minutes. Remove from oven and sprinkle with lemon juice before serving.

Nutrition Information: 110 calories, 4.5g fat, 10 mg cholesterol, 590mg sodium, 9g carbohydrate, 5g fiber, 11g protein

Exchanges: 0.5 Carbohydrate, 1.5 Protein, 1 Fat

Roasted Asparagus with New Potatoes

Makes 8 servings.

1 pound small red potatoes, cut into quarters

2 tablespoons olive oil

1 pound fresh asparagus, cut into 2 inch pieces

½ cup shallots, thinly sliced

1 teaspoon fresh thyme, chopped

½ teaspoon each salt and fresh ground pepper

2 teaspoons fresh lemon juice

1. Preheat oven to 425 degrees.

2. In large bowl, toss potatoes with olive oil. Spread potatoes on jelly roll pan.

3. Roast for 15 minutes; toss with spatula halfway through cooking time.

4. Remove from oven and add asparagus, shallots, thyme, and seasoning. Roast an additional 10 minutes or until asparagus is crisp tender.

5. Remove from oven, sprinkle with lemon juice, toss gently, and serve.

Nutrition Information: 190 calories, 7g fat, 0mg cholesterol, 310mg sodium, 28g carbohydrate, 4g fiber, 6g protein

Exchanges: 2 Carbohydrate, 1 Protein, 1 Fat

Asparagus has been celebrated for centuries as a natural diuretic. It is rich in asparagine, which increases urination and can clear the body of excess salts to reduce puffiness and swelling.

Roasted Brussels Sprouts

Makes 6 servings.

1 ½ pounds Brussels sprouts, stemmed, rinsed, and cut in half

3 tablespoons olive oil, divided

½ teaspoon each salt and fresh ground black pepper

1 tablespoon balsamic vinegar

1 teaspoon honey

1. Preheat oven to 425 degrees.
2. Rinse Brussels sprouts and cut in half; dry on paper towels. Place in single layer on large jelly roll pan.
3. Drizzle with 2 tablespoons of olive oil and season with salt and pepper. Roast for 20 minutes, stirring occasionally to ensure even browning.
4. Remove from oven and drizzle with remaining 1 tablespoon olive oil, balsamic vinegar, and honey. Toss gently and serve.

Nutrition Information: 130 calories, 7g fat, 0mg cholesterol, 220mg sodium, 12g carbohydrate, 4g fiber, 4g protein

Exchanges: 1 Carbohydrate, 0.5 Protein, 1 Fat

I like adding extra fresh ground black pepper just before serving to give an extra AI boost to this delicious cruciferous vegetable!

Sautéed Spinach

Makes 4 servings.

- 1 pound of spinach, stems removed
- 2 tablespoons olive oil
- 3 cloves garlic, thinly sliced
- ¼ teaspoon crushed red pepper flakes
- 1 teaspoon each salt and fresh ground black pepper
- 1 tablespoon balsamic vinegar

1. Bring large pot of water to boil over high heat. Add spinach all at once, stir, and drain immediately into colander. Place spinach on paper towels and press out as much liquid as possible.

2. To sauté, heat oil in large nonstick skillet. Add garlic and pepper flakes and sauté until garlic begins to turn golden, about 1 minute, stirring constantly to avoid burning.

3. Add spinach to skillet, stirring to coat with oil. Cook just until heated through, about 1 minute. Season with salt and pepper. Transfer to serving platter and drizzle with balsamic vinegar before serving.

Nutrition Information: 90 calories, 7g fat, 0mg cholesterol, 380mg sodium, 6g carbohydrate, 3g fiber, 3g protein

Exchanges: 0.5 Carbohydrate, 0.5 Protein, 1 Fat

Sweet Potato Fries

Makes 6 servings.

3 medium sweet potatoes, scrubbed clean

3 tablespoons olive oil

½ teaspoon each fresh cracked sea salt and fresh ground black pepper

1 tablespoon chopped fresh parsley

1. Preheat oven to 400 degrees.

2. Cut sweet potatoes into ½-inch thick strips. Place in large bowl and toss with olive oil.

3. Place on large jelly roll pan and roast for 15 minutes. Turn and roast another 15 minutes or until potatoes are browned and crispy.

4. Remove from oven and sprinkle with salt, pepper, and parsley before serving.

Nutrition Information: 130 calories, 7g fat, 0mg cholesterol, 220mg sodium, 17g carbohydrate, 2g fiber, 1g protein

Exchanges: 1 Carbohydrate, 0 Protein, 1 Fat

Zucchini, Yellow Squash & Tomato Packets

Makes 6 servings.

2 medium zucchini, sliced thin

2 medium yellow squash, sliced thin

1 medium sweet yellow onion, sliced thin

5 Roma tomatoes, sliced ¼-inch thick

2 tablespoons extra-virgin olive oil

½ teaspoon each salt and fresh ground black pepper

1 cup sharp low-fat cheddar cheese

¼ cup basil, chiffonade

1. Preheat grill or oven to 350 degrees.

2. In large bowl, combine zucchini, yellow squash, onion, and tomatoes. Drizzle with olive oil, season with salt and pepper and toss lightly.

3. Tear off a large piece of heavy duty aluminum foil. Spray foil with cooking spray and place vegetable mixture in center. Fold into a packet, leaving some space for air to circulate and allow for even cooking.

4. Grill over indirect heat (or place on cookie sheet in oven) for 7 minutes; then flip packet over and cook an additional 5-7 minutes.

5. Remove and let packet rest for 5 minutes before opening. Open packet, sprinkle with cheese and basil, and serve.

Nutrition Information: 110 calories, 6g fat, 5mg cholesterol, 370mg sodium, 9g carbohydrate, 3g fiber, 7g protein

Exchanges: 0.5 Carbohydrate, 1Protein, 1 Fat

I like to add 2 tablespoons of diced pickled jalapeños. Not only does it add flavor, it also greatly boosts the AI benefit of the veggies!

Apple Sweet Potato Casserole

Makes 8 servings.

3 medium sweet potatoes, peeled and cut into 1-inch cubes

2 medium apples, peeled and cut into 1-inch cubes

⅓ cup dried cranberries

2 tablespoons brown sugar

½ teaspoon cinnamon

¼ teaspoon salt

2 tablespoons butter, melted

¼ cup toasted pecans, coarsely chopped

1. Toss sweet potatoes, apples, and dried cranberries together in large bowl. Sprinkle with brown sugar, cinnamon, and salt. Drizzle with melted butter and toss gently.

2. Spray medium baking dish with cooking spray. Pour sweet potato mixture into baking dish. Cover with foil and bake at 350 degrees for 50 minutes. Uncover and sprinkle with toasted pecans. Return to oven and bake an additional 10 minutes.

Nutrition Information: 140 calories, 6g fat, 10mg cholesterol, 90mg sodium, 22g carbohydrate, 3g fiber, 1g protein

Exchanges: 1.5 Carbohydrate, 0 Protein, 1 Fat

Sweet potatoes are loaded with antioxidants, unmatched in Vitamin A, and are excellent sources of Vitamin C, potassium, and soluble fiber.

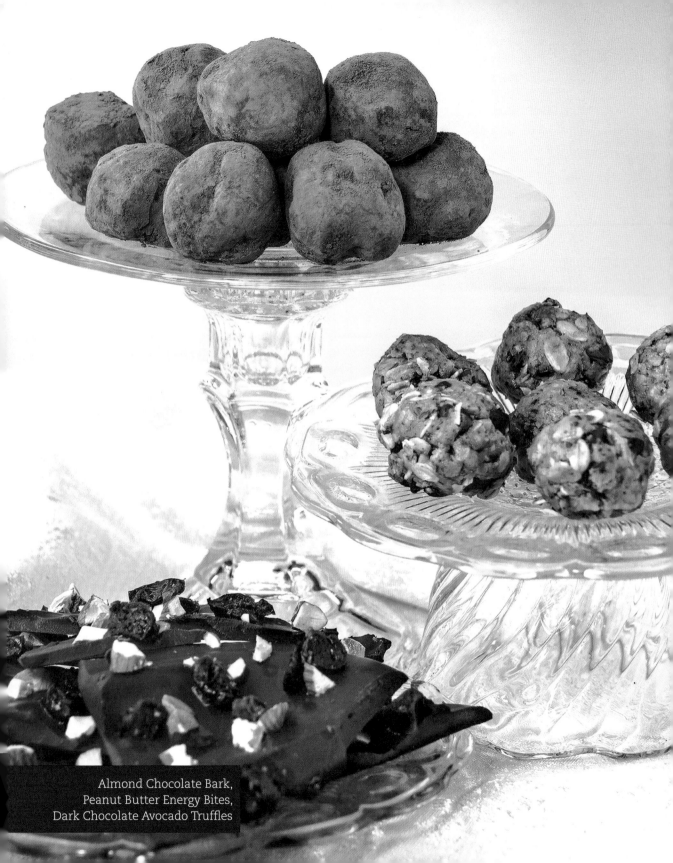

Almond Chocolate Bark,
Peanut Butter Energy Bites,
Dark Chocolate Avocado Truffles

Almond Chocolate Bark

Makes 36 servings.

Ingredients:

2 cups (11.5 oz.) extra dark chocolate chips (>70% cacao)

2 tablespoons chopped roasted almonds

2 tablespoons chopped dried cherries

Optional: sea salt

Directions:

1. Line 8 ½ × 12-inch baking sheet with parchment.

2. Melt chocolate chips by placing in microwave safe container. Microwave for 30 seconds and stir. Continue until just melted or about 1 ½ minutes total. Do not overcook!

3. Immediately spread in an even layer on baking sheet. Sprinkle chopped almonds and dried cherries over top and press lightly into the chocolate. Sprinkle sea salt on top, if desired.

4. Set aside until firm. Cut or break into 2-inch pieces to serve.

Nutrition Information: 50 calories, 4g fat, 0mg cholesterol, 0mg sodium, 4g carbohydrate, 1g fiber, 1g protein

Exchanges: 0.5 Carbohydrates, 0 Protein, 1 Fat

A small piece of dark chocolate is a delicious way to boost AI and take care of your sweet tooth at the same time!

• • •

Peanut Butter Energy Bites

Makes 20 servings.

½ cup natural peanut butter

⅓ cup honey

1 teaspoon vanilla extract

1 cup crispy rice cereal

⅔ cup toasted, unsweetened coconut flakes

½ cup protein powder

1 tablespoon ground flaxseed

½ cup mini morsel dark chocolate chips

¼ teaspoon cinnamon

1. Mix first three ingredients together in a medium bowl and add additional ingredients until thoroughly mixed. Cover and let chill in the refrigerator for 30 minutes.

2. Once chilled, using a tablespoon, scoop out individual bites and roll into balls. Store in an airtight container and keep refrigerated for up to 1 week.

Nutritional Information: 140 calories, 7g fat, 15mg cholesterol, 60mg sodium, 13g carbohydrate, 1g fiber, 7g protein

Exchanges: 1 Carbohydrate, 1 Protein, 1 Fat

Try this for a perfect complete snack giving you both the carbohydrate you need for quick energy and the healthy fat and protein you need for staying power!

• • •

Dark Chocolate Avocado Truffles

Makes 12 truffles.

6 ounces dark chocolate chips (>70% cacao)

⅓ cup mashed avocado

½ teaspoon vanilla extract

Pinch of salt

2 tablespoons cocoa powder

1. Place chocolate chips in medium glass bowl; microwave 30 seconds. Stir and microwave 15 seconds; stir until smooth.

2. Mash the avocado with a fork until no lumps are visible, then stir into the melted chocolate mixture until smooth. Stir in vanilla and salt. Place in the refrigerator to set for 20 minutes, or until slightly firm to the touch.

3. Remove mixture from the refrigerator and use a tablespoon to form chocolate into 12 balls. Place on pan lined with parchment paper. Working quickly, roll balls between the palms of your hands to create a smooth surface.

4. Place 2 tablespoons cocoa powder in small bowl and roll each truffle to coat. Serve immediately or store in the refrigerator.

Nutrition Information: 80 calories, 5g fat, 0mg cholesterol, 30mg sodium, 10g carbohydrate, 2g fiber, 1g protein

Exchanges: 0.5 Carbohydrate, 0 Protein, 1 Fat

Avocados are rich in monounsaturated fats, making them a powerful source of anti-inflammatory nutrition. They add a rich creamy texture to your favorite smoothie . . . or truffle!

Apple Oatmeal Cookies

Makes 4 dozen.

½ cup all-purpose flour

½ cup whole wheat flour

1 teaspoon baking soda

½ teaspoon salt

1 cup old-fashioned oats, uncooked

½ cup firmly packed brown sugar

1 teaspoon ground cinnamon

1 egg

½ cup canola oil

1 teaspoon vanilla extract

1 cup peeled, shredded apple

⅓ cup dried cranberries or raisins

⅓ cup chopped toasted pecans

1. Combine flours, baking soda, salt, oats, brown sugar, and cinnamon in a large bowl, mixing well.

2. In small bowl, whisk together egg, oil, and vanilla and stir into dry ingredients. Add shredded apple, raisins, and pecans, and stir until just blended.

3. Drop dough by rounded teaspoons onto greased cookie sheets. Bake at 350 degrees for 10-12 minutes or until golden brown. Carefully transfer cookies to wire racks to cool.

Nutrition Information (1 Cookie): 50 calories, 3g fat, 5mg cholesterol, 55mg sodium, 5g carbohydrate, 0g fiber, 1g protein

Exchanges: 0.5 Carbohydrate, 0 Protein, 0.5 Fat

Oats are a naturally gluten-free food high in soluble fiber. A diet rich in soluble fiber can improve cholesterol and moderate glucose levels.

Chocolate Almond Cranberry Crisps

Makes 36 crisps.

2 cups (11.5 oz.) dark chocolate chips (>70% cacao)

1 ½ cups crispy rice cereal

¾ cup unsweetened dried cranberries

⅓ cup slivered almonds

½ teaspoon vanilla

1. Cover large baking sheet with wax paper.

2. Place chocolate chips in medium glass bowl; microwave on high for 45 seconds. Stir and microwave an additional 45 seconds or until almost melted. Stir until smooth. Add cereal and remaining ingredients; stir quickly to combine.

3. Drop mixture by tablespoonfuls onto wax paper; chill 1 hour or until firm.

Nutrition Information (1 Crisp): 80 calories, 4.5g fat, 0mg cholesterol, 10mg sodium, 11g carbohydrate, 1g fiber, 1g protein

Exchanges: 1 Carbohydrate, 0 Protein, 1 Fat

Pavlova

Makes 6 servings.

3 egg whites, room temperature

¼ teaspoon cream of tartar

⅓ cup sugar, divided

½ teaspoon vanilla extract

3 cups mixed berries

1. Preheat oven to 175 degrees. Use the convection feature if you have it.

2. Line two cookie sheets with parchment paper.

3. Beat egg whites on medium speed until frothy. Add cream of tartar and increase speed to medium-high or high. When the egg whites have thickened and stiffened, sprinkle in one-half of the sugar and the vanilla. Continue to beat another minute to incorporate the sugar. You should have a stiff meringue that holds a peak. Remove from mixer and fold in the remaining sugar.

4. Spoon meringue evenly onto the cookie sheets in 6 mounds (about ¼ cup each). Use a spoon to form a depression in the middle of each mound to hold the fruit.

5. Bake until the meringues are dry and will separate from the parchment with a gentle nudge. This will take at least 90 minutes and may take as long as 4 hours, depending on the humidity. Note: If it is a very humid day, don't try to bake these. They'll be chewy, instead of dry and airy as they are intended to be. After they are done, turn off the oven and leave the meringues inside until cool (2-3 hours). You can store these in a zippered plastic bag or container for several days.

6. Top with berries and serve.

Nutrition Information: 70 calories, 0g fat, 0mg cholesterol, 25mg sodium, 16g carbohydrate, 3g fiber, 2g protein

Exchanges: 1 Carbohydrate, 0.5 Protein, 0 Fat

Cranberry Pumpkin Cookies

Makes 3 dozen.

½ cup butter, softened

¾ cup sugar

1 teaspoon vanilla extract

1 egg

1 cup canned pumpkin puree

1 ¼ cups all-purpose flour

1 cup whole wheat flour

2 teaspoons baking powder

1 teaspoon baking soda

½ teaspoon salt

1 teaspoon ground cinnamon

1 cup fresh cranberries, cut in half

1 tablespoon fresh orange zest

½ cup chopped walnuts

1. Heat oven to 375 degrees. Spray cooking sheet with cooking spray.

2. In large mixing bowl, cream together butter and sugar. Add vanilla, egg, and pumpkin. In separate bowl, blend together flours, baking powder, baking soda, salt, and cinnamon. Stir into pumpkin mixture until well blended.

3. Fold in cranberries, orange zest, and walnuts. Drop by teaspoonfuls onto cookie sheet.

4. Bake for 10-12 minutes or until golden brown.

Nutrition Information (1 cookie): 60 calories, 4g fat, 15mg cholesterol, 120mg sodium, 7g carbohydrate, 1g fiber, 1g protein

Exchanges: 0.5 Carbohydrate, 0 Protein, 1 Fat

Pumpkin is a delightful superfood loaded with beta-carotene, which can help do everything from discouraging kidney stones to subduing inflammation!

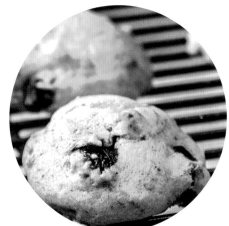

Cranberry Pumpkin Cookies

Meyer Lemon Budino (Italian Lemon Pudding)

Makes 6 servings.

½ cup sugar

3 large eggs, separated

¼ cup flour

¼ cup fresh Meyer lemon juice*

2 tablespoons fresh regular lemon juice

1 tablespoon fresh Meyer lemon zest

¾ cup low-fat milk

*If Meyer lemons are not available, use fresh orange or tangerine juice instead.

1. Preheat oven to 350 degrees. Measure sugar to ½ cup, then remove 2 tablespoons of sugar; set aside. Lightly butter 6 medium ramekins; set aside.

2. In medium bowl, combine sugar (all but 2 tablespoons), egg yolks, flour, both measures of lemon juice, and zest. Whisk until blended, then add milk and whisk again until well blended.

3. Using electric mixer, beat egg whites in medium bowl until frothy. Gradually add remaining 2 tablespoons of sugar and beat until soft peaks form.

4. Carefully fold the egg whites into the lemon mixture. Divide evenly between prepared ramekins. Place in roasting pan and add water into the pan up to depth of custard in cups. Carefully place in oven and bake for 30 minutes or until tops are golden and spring back when lightly touched.

5. Remove ramekins from water and serve warm or chilled.

Nutrition Information: 90 calories, 3g fat, 105mg cholesterol, 50mg sodium, 15g carbohydrate, 0g fiber, 4g protein

Exchanges: 1 Carbohydrate, 0.5 Protein, 0.5 Fat

Sweet Cherry Clafoutis

Makes 8 servings.

2 tablespoons melted butter

2 cups fresh cherries, pitted

3 large eggs, lightly beaten

1 cup low fat milk (at room temperature)

½ cup sugar

½ teaspoon fresh lemon zest

½ teaspoon each pure vanilla extract and almond extract

⅛ teaspoon salt

½ cup flour

1. Preheat oven to 375 degrees. Coat a 10-inch oven-proof skillet with melted butter. Arrange cherries in single layer in buttered skillet and set aside.

2. In medium bowl, combine eggs, milk, sugar, zest, extracts, and salt and whisk until smooth. Add flour and whisk just until combined. Pour over cherries in prepared skillet. Bake until set, puffed, and light golden brown around the edges, about 30 minutes.

3. Place pan on wire rack and let cool for 10 minutes. The clafoutis will deflate. Cut into wedges, serve warm for breakfast or dessert.

Nutrition Information: 120 calories, 5g fat, 90mg cholesterol, 100mg sodium, 15g carbohydrate, 1g fiber, 4g protein

Exchanges: 1 Carbohydrate, 0.5 Protein, 1 Fat

Cherries are an anti-inflammatory powerhouse; enjoy this delicious rustic French treat as a part of breakfast or for dessert.

Apple Granola Bites

Makes 8 servings.

2 medium honey crisp apples

4 tablespoons natural peanut butter

1 cup low-fat granola

⅓ cup dark chocolate chips (>70% cacao)

1. Cut apples into approximately 6 wedges each, removing cores.

2. Spread peanut butter on one side of each apple wedge.

3. Spread granola onto a plate and press the apple wedges, peanut butter side down, to cover.

4. Melt chocolate chips in microwavable bowl for 30 seconds. With spoon, drizzle melted chocolate over apples.

Nutrition Information: 150 calories, 7g fat, 0mg cholesterol, 65mg sodium, 23g carbohydrate, 3g fiber, 3g protein

Exchanges: 1.5 Carbohydrate, 0.5 Protein, 1.5 Fat

Chapter 5

Creating Your Personal Anti-Inflammatory Plan

*N*ow that you have a clear understanding of anti-inflammatory foods, and have seen the research indicating its power in preventing and/or managing chronic disease, it's time to create a plan of action!

In my years of practice, I have realized that there simply had to be more we could do to get out in front of chronic disease and give people the tools they need to help prevent it from happening in the first place. I set this out as a challenge to my brilliant team of professionals at JTA, and together, we have spent countless hours researching the data on anti-inflammatory foods and their positive impact on long-term health. From these findings, I have designed four easy-to-follow steps to give you a practical approach to making AI work for you. The steps listed on the next page will be discussed in detail in this chapter.

Step 1: Assess Your Need
Step 2: Assemble Your Helpful Anti-Inflammatory Tools
Step 3: Design Your Plan
Step 4: Execute Your Plan

Step 1: Assess Your Need

To begin, complete the simple Personal Inventory (PI) survey on page 54. It will help you gain perspective and insight on your need for making a healthy lifestyle change.

Step 2: Assemble Your AI Food Tools

Now that you have completed your personal inventory and have recognized where you need to make changes, it is important to gain a foundation of knowledge on why and how to get started. I've included practical tools throughout this section that will be helpful as you implement your new healthy lifestyle.

To build a realistic plan you can use, I've created an easy-reference AI Shopping List that appears after the Personal Inventory. Make copies, scan it into your phone—whatever gives you ready access to your shopping list of healthy food choices! A kitchen stocked with fresh, healthy food items is your best bet for consistently making healthy food choices.

In addition to including AI foods to build your pantry, there is an evolving area of research looking at the AI benefits of herbs and spices. I've included a list of the top AI herbs and spices for you to keep as a handy reference. Not only are these strongly anti-inflammatory in their own right, but many are known to enhance the bioavailability of other AI foods. Adding these herbs and spices to your favorite fruits and vegetables is a great way to get more

AI 'bang for your buck' without adding additional calories. Experiment freely with these flavor powerhouses to see how they may fit deliciously into your daily diet. It is best to purchase herbs in small quantities and replace them often, as they tend to lose their potency.

Step 3: Design Your Plan

Now that you have assembled your handy-dandy lists of foods, herbs, and spices to fight chronic inflammation, it is time for us to help craft a simple plan of action to build these into your daily life!

In addition to knowing the best foods to choose and those to avoid, I want to make sure you know the accepted guidelines for designing a healthy eating plan. The driving force for most of us who are seeking a healthier lifestyle is the desire to increase energy. When our bodies are under-fueled our energy is low, we lose focus, our productivity suffers, we feel fatigued, and our mood suffers. A healthy body is fueled and ready to embrace the day.

I have found that regardless of a person's diagnosis or health challenges, everyone can benefit from a refresher course on the basics of healthy eating. Misinformation bombards us about what is and is not healthy, and I find it is always helpful to define what science has to say about healthy eating. To do this, I have developed a set of six principles that help define how to fuel and train your body back to health. These principles appear on page 60.

• • •

Now that you know the basics, it is time to take a look at a sample meal plan that follows the six principles above while also including AI food selections. The sample plan is based on 1400 calories a day (see the end of this chapter).

If you would like to know your suggested calorie level and get a personalized meal plan from JTA, visit our website at www.jtawellness.com to join our lifestyle membership program. Includes access to monthly webcasts, online cooking classes, and audio podcasts.

As you design your plan, I would encourage you to take time to create a list of what you plan to eat for breakfast, lunch, and dinner, along with your morning, afternoon, and bedtime snacks. Include the time of day you will eat and make sure you have chosen items that fit in your lifestyle. If your job requires you to be in the car, you might want to choose nuts and a piece of fruit over Greek yogurt—unless you plan to buy a cooler for your car. The message here is to be practical and make your plan fit your lifestyle. If you try to deviate too much from your normal routine, it will be difficult to maintain.

Step 4: Execute Your Plan

Recognize this is a journey. Give yourself permission to not be perfect. Rest in the fact that you will learn every day how to execute your new AI lifestyle more efficiently and effectively as you continue to practice. The good news is, the more AI principles you can bring into your life, the better you will feel!

•   •   •

List the top five foods you plan to incorporate now as a part of the new "healthier" you.

1. _____

2. _____

3. _____

4. _____

5. _____

What three spices can I begin to include in foods I already enjoy that will increase anti-inflammatory absorption?

1. _____

2. _____

3. _____

Of Jan's Six Principles to Live By, what am I doing well? _____

_____

_____

Where do I need to improve? _____

_____

_____

The biggest challenge I face in converting to the AI lifestyle is _____

_____

_____

_____

After reading this chapter, the greatest opportunity I have for improving my nutrition is to _____

_____

_____

Eat Well to Be Well Personal Inventory

Circle the response that best describes you in each of the following questions.

Rank your current body weight.

-3 PI	-1 PI	+5 AI *	-2 PI	-5 PI
Significantly Underweight	10-15 lbs. under a healthy weight	Healthy Weight	10-15 lbs. over a healthy weight	Significantly Overweight

Which of the following describes any recent weight changes you have experienced?

-5 PI	-2 PI	+5 AI *	+2 AI	+5 AI
Gained 10% or more of my body weight	Gained a few pounds	Maintained a healthy body weight with little change	Intentionally lost a few pounds	Intentionally lost 10% or more of my body weight

In general, which of the following BEST describes your current diet?

-5 PI	-2 PI	+1 AI	+2 AI	+5 AI
I frequently eat: 1. foods high in sugar, refined carbs & animal fat 2. processed meat (bacon, ham, deli meat, sausage)	Several days a week, I eat: 1. foods high in sugar, refined carbs & animal fat 2. processed meat (bacon, ham, deli meat, sausage)	Mostly, I select: 1. a combination of carbs (complex & refined) and olive oil and/or canola oil 2. occasional processed foods with animal fat, sugar & refined carbs	I often: 1. eat whole grains, complex carbs & healthy oils (olive oil and/or canola) 2. limit processed foods with animal fat, sugar & refined carbs	I routinely: 1. select whole grains, complex carbs and healthy oils (olive oil and/or canola) 2. limit processed foods high in sugar & refined carbs

Which of the following BEST describes your current diet each day?

-5 PI	-2 PI	-1 PI	+2 AI	+5 AI
I typically eat fewer than two servings of fruits &vegetables	I eat a couple of servings of fruits & vegetables	I eat three to five servings of fruits & vegetables	I sometimes add fresh herbs and spices to meals and eat about five servings of fruits & vegetables	I often add fresh herbs and spices to meals and eat eight to ten servings of fruits & vegetables

How much active exercise do you do?

-5 PI	-2 PI	+1 AI	+2 AI	+5 AI
No regular physical activity	About 30 minutes a couple of times a week	At least 30 minutes most days	At least 45 minutes most days	At least 45 minutes most days & consistently active throughout the day

Which of the following BEST describes your sleep pattern on most nights?

-5 PI	-2 PI	+1 AI	+2 AI	+5 AI
Restless sleep and less than five hours	A little restless and less than six hours	Restless sleep for about eight hours	Sound sleep for about seven hours	Sound sleep for about eight hours

Do you use tobacco?

-5 PI	-2 PI	-1 PI	+2 AI	+5 AI
I use tobacco frequently	I use tobacco occasionally	I quit using tobacco less than six months ago	I quit using tobacco over five years ago	I have never used tobacco products

How would you describe your level of stress and anxiety on MOST days?

-5 PI	-2 PI	+1 AI	+2 AI	+5 AI
I am stressed and anxious every day and have difficulty controlling it	I am stressed and anxious many days and am challenged to control it	Stress is usually not a problem for me	I am engaged in activities I enjoy and successfully manage stress most days	I describe myself as thriving and engaged in activities I enjoy. I actively use techniques to manage stress and find balance in my life

How would you describe your oral health?

-5 PI	-2 PI	+1 AI	+2 AI	+5 AI
I have periodontal disease	I have inflamed gums and beginning stages of periodontal disease	My gums are healthy with no signs of periodontal disease	My gums are healthy and I see my dentist occasionally for preventive care	My gums are healthy and I see my dentist on a routine basis for preventive care.

Total AI (Anti-Inflammatory) Score _____

Total PI (Pro-Inflammatory) Score _____

Total (AI score - PI Score) _____

If your score is 35 to 45, you are an AI Rock Star!

If your score is 25 to 35, you have room for improvement, but are headed in the right direction.

If your score is 15 to 25, it is time to make some changes

If your score is below 15, be encouraged that by making significant changes in your lifestyle, good health is possible!

If your AI score is greater than your PI score, you are headed in the right direction. If PI is greater than AI, you've got some work to do! Now that you know your baseline, it is time to educate yourself on how to start making healthy changes. The more you can tip the balance to the anti-inflammatory side, the greater the rewards. You will quickly see how making small changes will make a huge impact on your health and well-being.

Anti-Inflammatory Shopping List

Non-starchy Vegetables
Serving size: unlimited
- ☐ Spinach
- ☐ Kale
- ☐ Swiss chard
- ☐ Mushrooms
- ☐ Cabbage
- ☐ Broccoli
- ☐ Brussels sprouts
- ☐ Cauliflower
- ☐ Onions
- ☐ Peppers
- ☐ Celery
- ☐ Carrots
- ☐ Cucumbers
- ☐ Green Beans
- ☐ Tomatoes
- ☐ Yellow Squash
- ☐ Zucchini

Fruits
Serving size: ¾–1 c or 1 small
- ☐ Apple
- ☐ Banana
- ☐ Blackberries
- ☐ Blueberries
- ☐ Cherries
- ☐ Grapes
- ☐ Grapefruit
- ☐ Kiwi
- ☐ Mango
- ☐ Melon
- ☐ Orange
- ☐ Papaya
- ☐ Peach
- ☐ Pear
- ☐ Pineapple
- ☐ Plum
- ☐ Raspberries
- ☐ Strawberries

Starchy Vegetables
Serving size: ½ cup
- ☐ Sweet potato
- ☐ Butternut squash
- ☐ Acorn squash
- ☐ Pumpkin
- ☐ Beans—black, garbanzo, lima, pinto, kidney, navy & white
- ☐ Peas—black-eyed and green peas
- ☐ Lentils

Grains
Serving size: ½–½ cup; 1 slice
- ☐ Brown rice
- ☐ Quinoa
- ☐ Couscous
- ☐ Bulgur wheat
- ☐ Whole grain pasta
- ☐ 100% whole grain bread (16 grams whole grain/serving)
- ☐ Oats—steel cut
- ☐ High fiber cereal (5 grams of bran/serving)

Protein
- ☐ Fish—wild caught, high in omega-3 such as salmon, albacore tuna, rainbow trout, black cod, & sardines
- ☐ Omega-3 fortified eggs
- ☐ Low-fat, natural cheese such as part-skim mozzarella & Parmesan
- ☐ Low-fat, unflavored Greek yogurt
- ☐ Low-fat cottage cheese
- ☐ Vegetable protein sources such as beans

- ☐ Soy foods such as tofu & tempeh
- ☐ Lean animal protein such as chicken or beef

Dairy
- ☐ Skim or 1% fat milk (1 cup/serving)
- ☐ Low-fat unflavored Greek yogurt (6 oz./serving)

Fat
- ☐ Olive oil
- ☐ Canola oil
- ☐ Avocados
- ☐ Nuts—especially walnuts, cashews, pumpkin seeds, almonds & nut butters made from these
- ☐ Black or green olives
- ☐ Ground flaxseed, chia seed, or hemp seed

Herbs and Spices
- ☐ Black pepper (whole & grind fresh when using)
- ☐ Cinnamon
- ☐ Clove (ground)
- ☐ Cumin
- ☐ Ginger (dried or fresh)
- ☐ Oregano (dried or fresh)
- ☐ Rosemary (dried or fresh)
- ☐ Turmeric (dried or fresh)

Treats
- ☐ >70% cacao dark chocolate (1 oz.)
- ☐ Red Wine

List of Anti-Inflammatory Herbs and Spices

Basil has potent anti-inflammatory effects from eugenol, which blocks the same enzyme as non-steroidal anti-inflammatory drugs; antioxidant flavonoids protect the body on a cellular level and contain oils that are effective antimicrobial substances.

Cardamom has essential oils with anti-inflammatory and anti-tumor properties.

Cayenne and all chili peppers contain capsaicinoids that have anti-inflammatory properties; cayenne has been shown to ease pain associated with arthritis and headaches.

Chamomile is an anti-inflammatory agent that can inhibit production of several pro-inflammatory substances in the body.

Chives are shown in research studies to have anti-inflammatory, antioxidant, and antimicrobial properties.

Cilantro & Coriander are anti-inflammatory and anti-microbial due to dodecenal; oils of the coriander plant are rich in phytonutrients.

Cinnamon is anti-inflammatory, antioxidant, and anti-microbial.

Garlic in lab studies is confirmed to be anti-inflammatory, may help prevent some types of cancer, and may help lower cholesterol.

Ginger has general anti-inflammatory properties, and may be beneficial in some neurodegenerative diseases.

Green Tea is an anti-inflammatory and anti-oxidant; the most important polyphenol in tea is EGCG (epigallocatechin gallate), which most likely provides cardiovascular and neurological benefits being reported in many studies; matcha is the most concentrated form.

Licorice is an herb that is rich in flavonoids, anti-inflammatory, and anti-microbial.

Marjoram is an herb that contains polyphenols known to be anti-inflammatory, antioxidant, and anti-microbial..

Nutmeg contains polyphenols that are anti-inflammatory and antioxidant.

Oregano is rich in polyphenols (possibly as much as 70 percent of the total oil) that are anti-inflammatory and antioxidant.

Parsley is an anti-inflammatory herb that is rich in polyphenols, vitamins, and minerals.

Pepper (black) is anti-inflammatory, anti-bacterial, and antioxidant; studies have shown that the chemical compounds of black pepper, particularly piperine, significantly increase the bioavailability of other nutrients.

Rosemary in several studies has shown anti-inflammatory effects due to flavonoids and rosmarinic acid.

Sage is rich in polyphenols and has been shown to be anti-inflammatory.

Thyme contains a phenol called carvacrol that suppresses the COX-2 gene much like resveratrol and provides anti-inflammatory benefits.

Turmeric contains curcumin, which is responsible for its strong anti-inflammatory effect.

Anti-Inflammatory Snacks on the GO!

Pick one from each column: Carbohydrate + Protein/Healthy Fat

Carbohydrate (Starch, Fruit, or Milk)	Protein/Healthy Fat
1 Small Apple	1 tablespoon Peanut Butter
2 tablespoon Raisins	16 Pistachios
8 Whole Wheat Pita Chips	2 tablespoons Olive Tapenade
1 oz >70% Cacao Dark Chocolate	10 Peanuts
1 Granola Bar	1 tablespoon Almond Butter
6 oz Fat-Free Yogurt	1 tablespoon Chia Seeds
1 cup Low-Fat Milk	1 Boiled Egg
3 cups Light Popcorn	6 Almonds
17 Red Grapes	6 Cashews
4 Melba Toast	1 oz Tuna
¼ cup Granola	4 Pecan Halves
1 Mini Whole-Wheat Bagel	1 oz Smoked Salmon (w/1 tablespoon of Fat-Free Cream Cheese + Red Onion)
1 ¼ cup Watermelon, diced	1 tsp Olive Oil + sprinkle Chili Powder & squeeze of Lime
½ cup Cooked Oatmeal	1 tablespoon Ground Flaxseed
15 Baked Tortilla Chips	2 tablespoons Guacamole
¾ cup Blackberries or Blueberries	1 tablespoon Pumpkin Seeds
1 slice Whole-Wheat Toast	2 Sardines in Mustard or Tomato Sauce
½ Whole Wheat English Muffin	1 tablespoon Cashew Butter
½ cup Veggie Sticks/Straws	8 Black Olives
1 cup Raspberries, frozen	¼ cup Cottage Cheese
8 Dried Apricots	1 tablespoon Sunflower Seeds
½ Whole Wheat Pita	1 teaspoon Tahini + sprinkle Cayenne Pepper + Raw Veggies (Cucumber, Peppers, Tomatoes, Red Onion, etc.)
1 ¼ cup Whole Strawberries	5 Hazelnuts
The following four items count as both carbohydrate and protein/healthy fat.	
4–6 oz Greek Yogurt	
⅓ cup Hummus	
½ cup Edamame	
½ cup Bean Dip	

Jan's Six Principles to Live By:

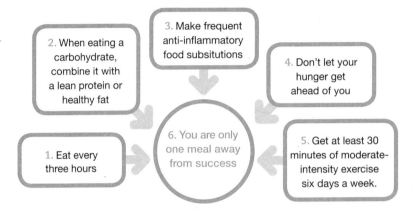

2. When eating a carbohydrate, combine it with a lean protein or healthy fat

3. Make frequent anti-inflammatory food subsitutions

4. Don't let your hunger get ahead of you

1. Eat every three hours

6. You are only one meal away from success

5. Get at least 30 minutes of moderate-intensity exercise six days a week.

1. Eat every three hours.

Our largest meal of the day takes about ninety minutes to two hours for our body to digest. If we are waiting more than three hours to eat again, we are asking our bodies to operate on no fuel. This is when our blood sugars begin to drop and we start to lose focus, productivity, and energy. The key to consistent metabolism and consistent energy is staying properly fueled.

2. When eating a carbohydrate, combine it with a lean protein or healthy fat.

Our body's first choice for energy is carbohydrate. We digest these very quickly, which can leave us feeling hungry and dissatisfied. Adding a protein or a healthy fat slows the digestion of the carbohydrate, leaving us feeling full longer and keeping our energy stable until it is time to eat again.

3. Make frequent anti-inflammatory food substitutions.

Many times when we are choosing what to eat, we are deciding between two foods from the same nutrient group, but one is a much better source of anti-inflammatory properties than the other. For example, if you are going to pan sauté a fish fillet, opt for olive oil rather than butter—same calories, similar taste, but much higher in AI benefits.

4. Don't let your hunger get ahead of you.

When we let ourselves get hungry, we tend to overeat, make bad food choices, or get hangry (so hungry we are angry)! To manage hunger, we must eat more frequently to keep our bodies fueled.

5. Get at least thirty minutes of moderate-intensity exercise six days a week.

If you are at a healthy weight, thirty minutes a day will help manage your weight. If you need to lose weight, the guideline is sixty minutes a day, six days a week. Studies are showing that any exercise greater than ten minutes can be cumulatively added to meet your daily goal.

6. You are only one meal away from success.

This is what I call my cheerleading statement! Deciding to change your lifestyle can be overwhelming. It is my goal to encourage you to understand that the only meal you need to get right is—your next one. The keys to adopting a healthy lifestyle that can be maintained for a lifetime are these:

- Be prepared with healthy, convenient items needed for meals and snacks.

- Have a Where, What, When plan for daily exercise.

- Execute your plan one meal, one day at a time.

Before you know it, thirty days will have passed. You will have lost a few pounds; you will notice a vast increase in your energy level; you will be ecstatic that you have lost weight without being hungry; and most importantly, this small taste of success will motivate you to continue.

1400 Calorie Sample Meal Plan

Breakfast

1 slice whole grain toast

¾ cup mixed berries

1 egg

Snack

1 small apple

1 tablespoon almond butter

Lunch

Spinach Salad with assorted chopped vegetables such as
carrots, broccoli, tomato, peppers, purple onion

2 oz diced chicken

5 whole grain crackers

1 medium pear

Snack

1 orange

1 low-fat string cheese

Dinner

Salmon (4 ounces) with fresh ground black pepper, dill, and lemon

Small sweet potato sprinkled with cinnamon

2 cups steamed broccoli and cauliflower

Snack

1 oz >70% cacao dark chocolate

6 almonds

*For a personalized meal plan based on your needs, contact JTA Wellness to
schedule an appointment with one of our Registered Dietitians*

Breakfast	Lunch	Dinner	Exercise
Carbohydrates: Choose 2			
1 Starch _____	1 Starch _____	2 Starches _____	_____
_____	_____	_____	_____
_____	_____	_____	_____
1 Fruit or Milk _____	1 Fruit _____	1 Fruit _____	_____
_____	_____	_____	_____
_____	_____	_____	_____
1 Protein _____	2 Proteins_____	_____	_____
_____	_____	3 Proteins _____	_____
_____	_____	_____	_____
0–1 Fat _____	1 Fat _____	_____	_____
_____	_____	1 Fat	_____
_____	_____	_____	_____
	0–1 Fat _____	_____	_____
	_____	_____	_____
	_____	2 Nonstarchy Vegetables_____	_____
		_____	_____
		_____	_____

Snack	Snack	Snack	Water
1 Starch, Fruit, or Milk _____	1 Starch, Fruit, or Milk _____	1 Starch, Fruit, or Milk _____	_____
_____	_____	_____	_____
1 Fat or Protein	1 Fat or Protein	1 Fat or Protein	_____
_____	_____	_____	_____
_____	_____	_____	_____

Chapter 6

Find Your Path to Fitness

You've probably heard the saying "You can't out-train a bad diet!" While I completely agree, I also believe the opposite of this saying is true—you can't take charge of your health by just changing your diet. It is virtually impossible to achieve your best health without finding your personal path to fitness. The path can be anything from swimming to tennis to walking, but it must be something!

I have many clients who have taken charge of their health using daily moderate exercise. One of my favorites is Garry. He walked into my office at his first appointment because his doctor had scared him into action by using the pre-diabetes word. Garry, like so many others, had been diagnosed years ago with an elevated cholesterol level that was managed with medication. At a follow-up appointment, his physician discovered high blood pressure, which led to additional medication. Now, this year's annual physical indicated elevated fasting glucose levels. His doctor referred him to my office in an effort to prevent adding yet another medication to manage his elevated blood sugars.

Here is a snapshot of Garry's health status at our initial appointment:

Weight: 286 pounds	Height: 5'10"	Age: 58	Fasting Glucose: 120	Hemoglobin A1C: 5.7

 Clinical note: what you may not know is this is an incredibly predictable scenario and one that we, as healthcare providers, see regularly. Our bodies want to stay healthy, but the inflammation that occurs from obesity, a sedentary lifestyle, and inflammatory food choices leads to health disparities. As we age, our body systems begin to wear. That, combined with a pro-inflammatory lifestyle, leads to health complications. The good news is that by taking action, these health issues are often reversible! By making the decision to decrease weight, eat healthy, and increase physical activity, it is possible to regain good health!

So picture this: Garry walks in, mad about his situation and mad that his doctor has sent him to see me. I had my work cut out for me to help him believe it was possible to make changes that could give him his health back!

As we began to talk, I asked him what would change if he could be healthy again. His answer was that he would not need so much medication. It turns out his biggest driving motivator for improved health was to get off medication and avoid adding new ones to fight diabetes. I used that desire to help him select small, manageable changes to ultimately reach his health goal. (I secretly suspected that once I could get him to see how much better he felt with a few dietary changes and moderate exercise, he'd be hooked!)

I was right! Garry has been working hard for the past nine months. He has learned to make healthier selections at the same restaurants he was enjoying before. He has an assortment of healthy snacks he enjoys at his desk throughout the day and is now walking 4 miles a day, six days a week. His energy is off the charts! He has lost sixty-six pounds and his physician has cut his cholesterol and blood pressure medication dosage in half. He has lost five inches in his waist circumference. His HgA1C is now 5.4 and fasting glucose is normal without medication.

Garry started with small changes to take charge of his health. The better he felt, the more changes he was willing to make. His significant lifestyle changes led to his reward—**he got his life back!**

We've long known that diet, exercise, and losing 5 to 10 percent of your body weight can improve cholesterol, blood pressure, and blood glucose numbers. Recent research is helping us understand that chronic inflammation may be responsible for those numbers being elevated in the first place. Garry's story is a wonderful example of how replacing pro-inflammatory with anti-inflammatory behaviors can dramatically improve health.

> Significant lifestyle changes lead to rewards— you can get your life back!

I'm often asked why adding physical activity is so important to improving health. As we age, if we've not been accustomed to being active, it is difficult to want to make the effort.

There are multiple reasons why getting adequate exercise is important to your good health.

1. Motion is the lotion for your joints. You've heard this old saying and it turns out to really be true. Research demonstrates over and over again the importance of staying active to reduce the aches and pains of arthritis and joint pain.

2. Movement acts as an anti-depressant. Aerobic exercise boosts oxygen circulation and spurs your brain to release feel-good chemicals called

endorphins. These combined with fresh air and sunshine can go a long way toward helping to elevate your mood.

3. Exercise improves stamina. When we are not accustomed to exercising, our bodies can get so stagnant that simply carrying a bag of groceries from the car to the house is taxing, leaving you out of breath and needing to sit down. Adding in exercise to build your endurance will give you increased stamina to make your tasks of daily living much easier to accomplish.

4. Exercise increases stability. Falls can lead to broken bones, which can lead to further complications and even death. By building stronger muscles, your body will be better equipped to recover its balance if you trip or have a misstep. This is such an important reason to add strength training.

5. Exercise builds lean muscle. The lean muscle mass gained from working out burns calories more efficiently, thus helping to better manage your weight.

6. Exercise helps manage stress. There is nothing more effective in helping to manage stress than a great workout! It is a healthy avenue for releasing frustrations. It lowers your blood pressure. It can be a wonderful time to sort through your thoughts and get a game plan for how best to handle difficult situations. It is funny how taking charge of your fitness can often bring confidence to handle other areas of your life.

7. Exercise increases metabolism. By exercising, we can turn up the heat on our metabolic flame. This allows our body to more efficiently burn the calories we consume.

If you're not active now, tell your health care provider you're going to start exercising—they'll root for you and make sure you are physically ready to get moving.

If you have not recently exercised, it is important to start slowly to avoid injury. Both sedentary behavior and excessive exercise can be harmful. Seek moderation and you will find the balance that is right for you. The ultimate goal is sixty minutes a day, six days a week for weight loss; thirty minutes a day, six days a week for weight maintenance.

For most people, a good daily walking plan is a safe, very effective way to start improving your health. It is a great stress reducer, it is very effective at managing your weight, and it helps stave off chronic inflammation.

If you are looking for a plan to get started, look no further! Here is a guide to walking your way to health!

•   •   •

What is stopping you from starting your path to fitness? _____

_____

_____

_____

What will you do to take your exercise to the next level? _____

_____

_____

_____

There will be days you don't feel like exercising. What will you do when you don't want to go? _____

_____

_____

_____

Walk Your Way to Good Health—
Thirty Days to a New You!

JTA has designed a walking plan for you! Follow this simple routine and you will be astonished at the results you see in thirty days! Our plan will boost your calorie burn by alternating a variety of walking routines—everything from moderately paced jaunts to high-speed intervals. You will want to start and finish each of your workouts with five minutes of slow walking to warm up and cool down.

Easy Walk—Monday, Wednesday & Friday

It's easy because you really will not be pushing yourself hard. The goal is to walk at a pace that you might use if you were running late to an appointment. You should feel a slightly elevated heart rate.

Week 1: 30 minutes

Week 2: 35 minutes

Week 3: 40 minutes

Week 4: 45 minutes

Interval Walk—Tuesday & Thursday

Here's where you will pick up the pace—and your calorie burn—for about 30 to 90 seconds before slowing down to catch your breath. During the speed interval, you should be walking so that you're breathing hard.

Week 1: 5 minutes at moderate pace, 30-second speed interval.
Repeat 4 times = 22 minutes

Week 2: 5 minutes at moderate pace, 60-second speed interval.
Repeat 4 times = 24 minutes

Week 3: 5 minutes at moderate pace, 90-second speed interval.
Repeat 4 times = 26 minutes

Week 4: 5 minutes at moderate pace, 60-second speed interval.
Repeat 5 times = 30 minutes

Speed Walk—Saturday

Pick an easy-to-remember route that will take about 30 minutes to complete at a fast pace. Each week, try to cover the same distance in less time.

Long Walk—Sunday

This is your endurance workout. Walk at a pace you can comfortably sustain for the recommended time. Focus on enjoying your walk, not on your pace.

Week 1: 45 minutes

Week 2: 50 minutes

Week 3: 55 minutes

Week 4: 60 minutes

Chapter 7

Strategies for Managing Stress

Change is a part of life—some changes are welcomed and some simply endured. Regardless, any kind of change—good or bad—can be stressful.

Stress can be defined as that feeling you have when you are faced with more or different challenges than you are accustomed to handling. When you are stressed, your body responds as though you were in danger. It produces hormones that speed up your heart, make you breathe faster, and give you a burst of energy. This is known as the fight-or-flight stress response. From a nutrition perspective, stress usually affects people in one of two ways. You may be either a "stress eater" or you lose your appetite.

> Any kind of change—good or bad—can be stressful.

Recurrent stress can have harmful effects and is one of the main contributors to chronic inflammation. It can be linked to headaches, gastrointestinal disorders, back and shoulder pain, and trouble sleeping. It can weaken your immune system, making it harder to fight off disease. If you are already dealing with a health problem, stress can make it worse, often making you moody, tense, or depressed.

One of the by-products of stress is the feeling that your life is out of control. While our first response might involve inhaling a bag of Oreo cookies, I've found a healthier approach is to take a step back, analyze what is really going on, and make some changes that will help bring order and stability back to your life—and thus help reduce your stress. Here are some areas you may want to consider.

Simplify

When things are going well, we are usually pretty good at multi-tasking, but when things get stressful, it is overwhelming to try to take care of everything on our plate. This is the time to take a step back, determine your priorities, and learn to say no. This decision will make you feel better. You will begin to feel you are gaining control over certain areas of your life, and by saying no you may just be giving someone else an opportunity to shine! One of my clients recently gave me a very wise example of simplifying life to help manage her stress. She has always been very active in her church—you know this giving type of person—any time they needed a Sunday School class taught, an event planned, a Vacation Bible School teacher, someone to work the nursery, she always said yes. Suddenly, she was given a bad health diagnosis, her daughter and grandbaby moved back home, she was still working a very busy job, and life was chaos. She knew it was time to simplify and give herself time to deal with her immediate life

> This is the time to take a step back, determine your priorities, and learn to say no.

challenges. She resigned from everything that she could, took time to take care of herself and her family, and gave others the opportunity to step in. Simplifying your life in a time of stress can be most helpful in maintaining and keeping your mental and physical health.

Declutter

Often when we get stressed, we begin to let everything else go. Our house, closets, drawers, desks, and cars look like a bomb went off. By deciding to take control of one small area at a time, you will be shocked at how much better you feel. Small example: Bruce and I had a second desk in the office off of our kitchen. I don't like clutter on the island, so instead we would go around the corner and pile mail, books, newspaper clippings, etc., on this desk. It was such an eyesore! One weekend I said, "Why don't we get rid of that desk? It is so cluttered no one can even use it. I don't think we'd ever miss it!" So we cleaned it off and took it out of the office. Bruce and I both find ourselves walking into the office going, "WOW, this looks so much better. I feel like I could work in here again! Sure glad we got that done! Feels like we have our office back!" One small task that took a couple of hours to do, but it made such a difference! We felt a sense of accomplishment—like we had taken charge of our mess and fixed it! Now instead of a place of chaos, it is a refuge.

> By deciding to take control of one small area at a time, you will be shocked at how much better you feel.

Relax

Taking downtime is so important to good health. Your downtime can be active or passive rest. Some people feel better after a round of golf or a game of tennis. Others need sit and stare time. Actually, you need both. Give yourself permission to be active with others and to be alone to reflect and regenerate.

Sleep

Poor sleep is pro-inflammatory and can really play havoc with your good health. If getting good sleep is difficult for you, there is an entire chapter in this book with practical ideas on to how to improve your sleep. Be encouraged—there are numerous steps you can take to improve the quality of your sleep.

Stress-Busting Foods

Foods can help tame stress in several ways. Comfort foods, like a bowl of warm oatmeal, boost levels of serotonin, which is known to be an important brain-calming chemical. Other foods can cut levels of cortisol and adrenaline, which are stress hormones that take a toll on the body over time. Developing a healthy diet can counter the impact of stress by shoring up the immune system and lowering blood pressure.

Stress is a fact of life

Our goal should be to help manage stress so that it does not negatively affect our good health. Setting good personal boundaries is key to avoiding unnecessary stress. Perhaps Reinhold Niebuhr summarizes it best in the age-old Serenity Prayer:

God grant me the serenity
To accept the things I cannot change;
Courage to change the things I can;
And wisdom to know the difference.

● ● ●

What are the areas of your life you need to simplify or declutter to better manage your stress? _____
_____
_____

What will you do NOW to start taking time to relax? _____
_____
_____

Do you know which foods are stress busters?

Complex Carbohydrates. All carbohydrates prompt the brain to make more serotonin. For a steady supply of this feel-good chemical, it's best to eat complex carbs, which are digested more slowly. Good choices include whole grain breakfast cereals, breads, and pastas, as well as old-fashioned steel cut oatmeal.

Oranges. Oranges make the list for their wealth of vitamin C. Studies suggest this vitamin can curb levels of stress hormones while strengthening the immune system. In one study of people with high blood pressure and elevated cortisol (a stress hormone) levels, both conditions normalized more quickly when they took vitamin C before a stressful task.

Spinach. Popeye never lets stress get the best of him—maybe it's all the magnesium in his spinach! Too little magnesium may trigger headaches and fatigue, compounding the effects of stress. One cup of spinach goes a long way toward replenishing magnesium stores. Not a fan of spinach? Try kale or other green leafy vegetables, edamame, nuts, and salmon, which are also high in magnesium.

Fatty Fish. Omega-3 fatty acids, found in fish such as salmon and tuna, can prevent surges in stress hormones and may help protect against heart disease, depression, and PMS. For a steady supply of feel-good omega-3s, put fatty fish on your menu at least twice a week.

Black Tea. Drinking black tea may help you recover from stressful events more quickly. One study compared people who drank four cups of tea daily for six weeks with people who drank another beverage. The tea drinkers reported feeling calmer and had lower levels of the stress hormone cortisol after stressful situations.

Pistachios. Pistachios, as well as other nuts and seeds, are good sources of healthy fats. Eating a handful of pistachios, walnuts, or almonds every day may help lower your cholesterol, ease inflammation, make diabetes less likely, and help protect you against the effects of stress. Don't overdo it, though; nuts are rich in calories.

Avocados. One of the best ways to reduce high blood pressure is to get enough potassium. Most of us think of bananas when reaching for a potassium boost, but did you know avocado is also an excellent source of potassium? Guacamole is a healthy alternative when stress has you craving a high-fat treat.

Almonds. Almonds are chock-full of helpful vitamins: vitamin E to bolster the immune system, plus B vitamins, which may make you more resilient during bouts of stress and depression.

Raw Veggies. Crunchy raw vegetables can help ease stress in a purely mechanical way. Munching celery or carrot sticks helps release a clenched jaw and helps ward off tension.

Bedtime Snack. Carbs at bedtime can speed the release of serotonin and help you sleep better. Since heavy meals before bed can trigger heartburn, stick to something light, such as whole grain toast with a light spread of almond butter.

Milk. Another bedtime stress buster is the time-honored glass of milk. Research shows that calcium eases anxiety and mood swings linked to PMS. Dietitians typically recommend skim or low-fat milk.

Chapter 8

Tools for a Better Night's Sleep

*S*leep difficulties are one of the most common complaints I hear from clients. The CDC estimates that problems going to sleep or staying asleep affect from fifty to seventy million US adults. If you are having issues with sleep, you are not alone!

While poor-quality sleep is mostly an inconvenience, researchers from the University of Arizona have found a connection between persistent insomnia and increased inflammation and mortality. The study was published in *The American Journal of Medicine* and can be read by going to this link: www. jtawellness.com/insomnia

Many times, poor sleep is rooted in a physical condition that can be corrected, such as hormone imbalance or sleep apnea. If you are struggling with chronic sleep deprivation, it is time to have a complete physical to ensure you have eliminated all physical roadblocks that might be standing in the way of you and a restful night's sleep. Your physical may be followed by a complete sleep study if your physician feels it is warranted. Be sure to have the study done at an accredited sleep disorder center. To find one nearest you, go to www.sleepeducation.com/find-a-facility.

If you think you may be suffering from sleep issues, here is a quick 5-question quiz to help predict if further evaluation may be needed:

How do you know if you are sleep deprived?

1. Does a warm room, boring meeting, heavy meal, or low dose of alcohol make you drowsy?

2. Do you fall asleep within five minutes of getting into bed?

3. Do you need an alarm clock to wake up?

4. Do you hit the snooze button repeatedly?

5. Do you sleep extra hours on weekends?

Answer yes to two or more of these questions and consider yourself sleep deprived!

Whether or not you have physical reasons for poor sleep, there are steps to take to help get a better night's rest. Here are some tips you might consider to help improve your sleep.

5 Tips for a Better Night's Sleep

1. Watch your food and drink. Limit your quantity and your choices as bedtime approaches. Don't go to bed too hungry or too stuffed; both could interfere with sleep quality. Consume the majority of your daily fluid requirement (the recommended guideline is half your body weight in ounces) by late afternoon to make sure you are not hopping up and down all night going to the bathroom. Avoid caffeine after midday, because it is a stimulant and may contribute to sleep problems. Avoid alcohol within three hours of bedtime. Alcohol in excess can help you go to sleep quickly, but it often causes you to wake during the night and not be able to go back to sleep.

2. Establish a bedtime ritual. Turn off all electronics at least one hour before bed or wear blue daylight spectrum-blocking glasses, which may be purchased at www.litebook.com. Have a light snack such as ½ cup of Greek yogurt; take a hot shower or bath; read something enjoyable until you begin to get sleepy; then turn out the lights and go to sleep. Make sure you go to bed at approximately the same time every night and get up about the same time every morning Monday through Monday including weekends. The goal is to follow the same ritual so that your body recognizes, *Oh, I get it; when we do this we are getting ready to sleep!* We have one biological clock (one circadian rhythm); not one for the workweek and one for weekends. We need to synchronize the hours we feel sleepy with the hours we spend in bed.

3. Create a positive sleep environment. Have the room cool and dark. Choose a comfy pillow, one that holds your head, neck, and spinal cord in a straight line as if you were standing up. Choose a pillow that is

commensurate with where you begin your night (side, back, or stomach). Choose the right number of covers, and cozy pajamas, so you won't get tangled up during the night. If you need a sound machine or a fan, set that up. Remember: no TV, Internet, or phone for at least one hour before bedtime.

4. Get physical! Regular exercise will make an amazing difference in your quality of sleep. Make sure you are active thirty to sixty minutes a day.

5. Manage stress. The busyness of life and the stresses that accompany our crazy schedules often lead to sleepless nights. This is why step three is so important! Don't remind your brain of all you have to do the next day by checking emails as you turn out the lights! Jot down all of your worries on a notepad just before going to sleep so that you won't wake in the middle of the night when you can't do anything about them anyway. If something does come to your mind during the night, preventing you from going back to sleep, have your notepad handy, jot it down, and vow to deal with it in the morning!

A good night's sleep is critical to good health. It calms chronic inflammation, improves our mood, and increases our energy and our ability to deal with life challenges. Think how different your life could be if you got seven to eight hours of quality sleep!

●　●　●

What are the biggest roadblocks to a good night's sleep for you? _____

_____

_____

_____

What three things are you willing to try for one week to improve your sleep?

1. _____

2. _____

3. _____

Many thanks to Dr. James B. Maas for his contribution to this chapter. He is a former professor, department chair in psychology, and Stephen H. Weiss Presidential Fellow at Cornell University. He is well known as the author of *Sleep for Success!*, the gold standard for insight and strategies to guide you to a great night's sleep.

Chapter 9

Putting It All Together

To embrace anti-inflammatory living, we've covered multiple diet, exercise, and lifestyle changes that need to be addressed. Remember, with AI, the more positive changes you make, the more health improvement you will experience. The choice on what and how much to change is up to you.

In this book, we have discussed several changes that you can make to decrease chronic inflammation. By eliminating pro-inflammatory foods and adding in more AI foods, herbs, and spices, you should really start to notice that your inflammatory symptoms are diminishing. Combining diet and exercise with improved gut health, so that more nutrients can be absorbed from the awesome foods you are choosing, is a huge step toward reclaiming your good health. Add in getting a grip on your stress and learning to value sleep by

The more positive changes you make, the more health improvement you will experience.

creating a healthier sleep environment, and you will be well on your way to a healthier, happier, more rested you!

●   ●   ●   .

Let me pull all this together by telling you about one of my clients who I think has done an amazing job of reclaiming her health in the midst of some pretty tough challenges. As a clinician, I have the opportunity to observe people who are not feeling their best on a daily basis. Some are more motivated than others to do whatever it takes to feel better.

Gloria is a perfect example of someone who came in willing to fight for her health. She came to me about two years ago as a referral from her physician. She was suffering from debilitating dizziness; severe allergies to medications, chemicals, foods, and preservatives; and many other environmental allergies. She also was battling chronic migraines, Meniere's disease, chronic fatigue, and arthritis. She was unable to do much except lie around the house, nap two or three times a day, take multiple high-dose medications, and eat whatever she could that did not make her symptoms worse. She rarely left the house except for doctor appointments.

The first time I met Gloria I immediately noticed her ashen skin tone, her puffy face, and that she was so weak I could barely hear her when she tried to speak. Her husband, Ralph, accompanied her to the appointment and he has been at every appointment since. I believe his kind, caring support has been a huge part of Gloria's recovery.

We worked with Gloria on a meal plan to help avoid her long list of trigger foods and we encouraged her to eat more often throughout the day and include protein to give her improved strength and satiety. After several months we began to see some improvement, but still none of us were completely satisfied with the progress. I re-evaluated her list of medications and her list of illnesses, and at her next appointment told her I wanted to try something new—I wanted to try her on the FODMAP diet. This is the diet limiting high-fructose foods discussed in Chapter 3. In patients who are unable to properly digest these foods, eliminating them from the diet can be life-changing.

Since being on this diet, Gloria has made huge progress in her quest to get her health back. She is sleeping well at night and not napping at all during the day. Today, her skin color is good and her smile is bright. Thankfully, her migraines are managed, her energy has returned, and her dizziness from Meniere's disease is much improved. She is now able to attend church again, go shopping, enjoy light exercise, and do some traveling, all of which were completely out of the question prior to changing her diet.

> **Never give up hope of finding a solution.**

The message in Gloria's story is that she never gave up hope of finding a solution. She persistently kept coming back session after session, doing everything I asked of her, until we uncovered her path back to wellness. The determination I see in successful clients like Gloria motivates me and is a core source of the joy I find in being a health-care professional. I am inspired by their persistence to keep trying and never give up hope! They patiently implement their plan and do whatever it takes until they achieve the best health possible for them.

 If you'd like to see Gloria tell her story, visit our website at www.jtawellness.com/gloria. She has a powerful message about the difference the anti-inflammatory lifestyle has made in her quality of life.

Whether your goal is to do whatever it takes to prevent chronic inflammation and avoid chronic disease, or if you are already battling against disease that has been brought on by inflammation, I want you to know that good health is possible. It takes time, effort, dedication, and determination, but the reward of a long, healthy, happy life is SO worth your investment!

Throughout this book I've given you helpful tools and techniques to assist you in making anti-inflammatory living a practical, viable option for you. The recipe section of this book gives you over one hundred of my favorite anti-inflammatory recipes developed over my years as a foodie, dietitian, mom, wife, and dinner party guru. It is important to me that the food I serve and enjoy promotes health, but it is even more important to me that it is quick to fix and tastes amazing! I think you will find all of this to be true in the recipes I have included.

Bon Appétit!

Appendix

Research Studies on Inflammation, Diet, and Chronic Disease

A Review of Chronic Inflammation

Chronic inflammation is involved in the development and progression of degenerative diseases. As such, research into the effect of dietary habits on markers of inflammation is increasing rapidly. Markers of inflammation (C-reactive protein, Interleukin-6, and tumor necrosis factors) are measured in an attempt to understand how dietary interventions affect inflammation. The authors of this review found that most studies show significant benefits from anti-inflammatory dietary changes.

This review found that dietary glycemic load, glycemic index, fiber, fatty acid composition, magnesium, carotenoids, and flavonoids can affect inflammation. A diet style high in monounsaturated fats and fruits, vegetables, legumes, and grains has shown anti-inflammatory effects when compared with typical North American and Northern European dietary patterns.

Galland, L., "Diet and Inflammation." *Nutrition in Clinical Practice* 25, 6 (2010): 634-640.

Cancer

Chronic inflammation is an important factor in the development of colon cancer. This study was designed to investigate the association between dietary inflammatory index (DII) and colorectal cancer. The DII score for each participant was obtained from a dietary history questionnaire and known inflammatory properties of foods. Changes in genes associated with colorectal cancer were analyzed. Overall, high inflammatory diets are associated with increased risk of colorectal cancer. Dietary-related inflammation plays an important role in colorectal cancer development; thus, reducing inflammatory impact of foods we eat may help prevent development of colorectal cancer.

Zamora-Ros, R., Shivappa, N., Steck, S.E., Canzian, F., Landi, S., Alonso, M.H., Hébert, J.R., and Moreno, V. "Dietary Inflammatory Index and Inflammatory Gene Interactions in Relation to Colorectal Cancer Risk in the Bellvitge Colorectal Cancer Case-control Study." *Genes and Nutrition* 10. 1 (2015): 447.

Cancer

A team of researchers has found that dietary lipids, called sphingolipids, may provide a link between diet, inflammation, and cancer. A study reported in the *Journal of Clinical Investigation* provides evidence that a substance (sphingosine) produced by normal human cells can cause inflammation of the colon, inflammatory bowel disease (IBD), and inflammation-associated colon cancer. Plant-based soy sphingolipids may protect against these conditions. This study shows a direct link between diet, inflammation, and cancer.

Degagné, E., Pandurangan, A., Bandhuvula, P., Kumar, A., Eltanawy, A., Zhang, M., Yoshinaga, Y., Nefedov, M., De Jong, P. J., Fong, L.G., Young, S.G., Bittman, R., Ahmedi, Y., and Saba, J.D. "Sphingosine-1-phosphate Lyase Downregulation Promotes Colon Carcinogenesis through STAT3-activated MicroRNAs." *Journal of Clinical Investigation* 124, 12 (2014): 5368-384.

Cancer

Researchers examined the impact of multiple "metabolic syndrome" conditions (such as obesity, high blood pressure, elevated fasting glucose, etc.) on prostate cancer risk. Data showed the presence of two or more conditions was associated with an increased risk of high-grade disease. According to this study, diet and lifestyle may affect the risk of being diagnosed with prostate cancer. A healthy lifestyle may be a good first line of defense against being diagnosed with a life-threatening prostate cancer.

American Urological Association. "Metabolic Syndrome Disorders, Diet may Boost Prostate Cancer Risk." *Medical News Today*. June 20, 2015. http://www.medicalnewstoday.com/releases/277070.php

Cancer

New research suggests that an anti-inflammatory compound makes cancer cells mortal again by removing their ability to avoid programmed cell death. A compound (apigenin) found in parsley, celery, chamomile tea, and many other fruits and vegetables can stop breast cancer cells from inhibiting natural, programmed cell death. This study shows a potential cancer prevention strategy directly related to diet.

Ohio State University. "Compound In Mediterranean Diet Makes Cancer Cells 'Mortal'." *Medical News Today*. MediLexicon, Intl., May 23, 2013. Web. Accessed June 16, 2015. http://www.medicalnewstoday.com/releases/260826.php

Cardiovascular Disease and Diabetes

A systematic review of studies on the effect of the Mediterranean diet in diabetes control and cardiovascular risk was discussed. Data revealed the Mediterranean diet improved glycemic control and cardiovascular disease.

Sleiman, D., Al-Badri, M.R., and Azar, S.T. "Effect of Mediterranean Diet in Diabetes Control and Cardiovascular Risk Modification: A Systematic Review." *Frontiers in Public Health* 3, 69 (2015).

Cardiovascular Disease

Authors of this review article concluded that evidence indicates the intake of vegetables, nuts, and a Mediterranean-style diet is protective against cardiovascular disease. Intake of trans-fatty acids, unhealthy animal fats, and high-glycemic foods are harmful. Although the interventions varied across the studies, the overall conclusion is that diet is strongly associated with cardiovascular disease.

Mente, A., DeKoning, L., Shannon, H.S., and Anand, S.S. "A Systematic Review of the Evidence Supporting a Causal Link Between Dietary Factors and Coronary Heart Disease." *Archives of Internal Medicine* 169, 7 (2009): 659-69.

Cardiovascular Disease and other Inflammatory Diseases

Pro-inflammatory diets high in refined starches, sugar, and saturated and trans-fatty acids, and low in fruits, vegetables, whole grains, and omega-3 fatty acids may trigger chronic inflammation. Diets high in olive oil, fruits, vegetables, cereals, nuts and seeds; moderate in wine (with meals) and in consumption of fish, seafood, yogurt, cheese, poultry, and eggs; and low in consumption of red meat and processed meat characterize the Mediterranean style of eating. Several studies reviewed here conclude that this style of eating protects us against cancer, diabetes, obesity, atherosclerosis (by preventing formation of plaque in blood vessel walls), metabolic syndrome, and cognition disorders, all of which are associated with chronic inflammation.

Casas, R., Sacanella, E., and Estruch, R. "The Immune Protective Effect of the Mediterranean Diet against Chronic Low-grade Inflammatory Diseases." *Endocrine, Metabolic & Immune Disorders—Drug Targets* 14, 4 (2014): 245-54.

Cardiovascular Disease

"Reducing the incidence of coronary heart disease with diet is possible." Anti-inflammatory diet strategies include increased intake of omega-3 fatty acids, lower intake of saturated and trans fats, and higher amounts of fruits, vegetables, nuts, and whole grains, and lower amounts of refined grains. This review examines evidence about diet and inflammation. Diets that are high in refined starches, sugar, and saturated and trans-fatty acids; lack natural antioxidants and fiber from fruits, vegetables, and whole grains; and are low in omega-3 fatty acids cause chronic inflammation. Choosing healthy sources of carbohydrate, fat, and protein; engaging in regular physical activity; and refraining from smoking can protect against chronic disease. The typical "Western diet warms up inflammation, while healthy diets cool it down."

Giugliano, D., Ceriello, A., and Esposito, K. "The Effects of Diet on Inflammation." *Journal of the American College of Cardiology* 48, 4 (2006): 677-85.

Cardiovascular Disease

Review article of 147 studies involving diet and cardiovascular disease. Compelling evidence suggests three dietary strategies are effective to prevent cardiovascular disease: substitute non-hydrogenated unsaturated fats for saturated and trans fats; increase consumption of omega-3 fatty acids from fish, fish oil supplements, or plant sources; and consume a diet high in fruits, vegetables, nuts, and whole grains and low in refined grain products. Together with regular physical activity, avoidance of smoking, and maintaining healthy body weight, these dietary strategies may prevent cardiovascular disease.

Hu, F., and Willett, W. "Optimal Diets for Prevention of Coronary Heart Disease." *Journal of American Medical Association* 288, 20 (2002): 2569.

Chronic Kidney Disease

Markers of chronic inflammation in the blood were reduced in chronic kidney disease patients when white wine and olive oil were added to the diet.

Migliori, M., Panichi, V., De la Torre, R., Fitó, M., Covas, M., Bertelli, A., Muñoz-Aguayo, D., Scatena, A., Paoletti, S., and Ronco, C. "Anti-inflammatory Effect of White Wine in CKD Patients and Healthy Volunteers." *Blood Purification* 39, 1-3 (2015): 218-23.

Cognitive Decline

The intervention in this study is a personalized program based upon the disease process involved in Alzheimer's patients. Multiple lifestyle interventions provided dramatic "metabolic enhancement for neurodegeneration (MEND)." Ten people involved in the study included patients with Alzheimer's disease (AD) and those with other cognitive impairments. Nine of the ten achieved improvement in cognition in three to six months. The only exception was a patient with late-stage Alzheimer's. These improvements continued for two and one-half years from initial treatment. Therefore, a larger study is warranted. Further, the results may mean that early-stage cognitive decline may be stopped or even reversed with dietary intervention.

Bredesen, Dale E. "Reversal of Cognitive Decline: A Novel Therapeutic Program." *Aging* 6, 9 (2014): 707-717.

Depression

Depression is associated with chronic inflammation. This review article explores the role of inflammation and oxidative stress as possible mediators of depression. The sources of chronic inflammation that are linked to depression are psychosocial stressors, poor diet, physical inactivity, obesity, smoking, altered gut permeability, allergies, poor dental hygiene, sleep problems, and vitamin D deficiency. Some of these sources of inflammation may play a role in bipolar disorder, schizophrenia, autism, and post-traumatic stress disorder.

Berk, M., Williams, L., Jacka, F., O'Neil, A., Pasco, J., Moylan, S., Allen, N., Stuart, A., Hayley, A., Byrne, M., and Maes, M. "So Depression is an Inflammatory Disease, but Where Does the Inflammation Come From?" *BMC Medicine* 11, 200 (2013).

Diabetes

This study was designed to determine if a pistachio-rich diet reduces the prediabetes stage. Fasting glucose, insulin, and insulin resistance decreased significantly after the pistachio diet. Data suggest that pistachios are anti-inflammatory and lower glucose and insulin. Thus, this dietary intervention can reverse certain metabolic harmful effects of prediabetes.

Hernández-Alonso, P., Salas-Salvadó, J., Baldrich-Mora, M., Juanola-Falgarona M., and Bulló, M. "Beneficial Effect of Pistachio Consumption on Glucose Metabolism, Insulin Resistance, Inflammation, and Related Metabolic Risk Markers: A Randomized Clinical Trial." *Diabetes Care* 37, 11 (2014): 3098-105.

Inflammatory Bowel Disease (IBD)

IBD is a chronic disease associated with chronic inflammation. Turmeric has been used over several centuries to treat inflammatory disorders. We found that a turmeric extract reduced so-called "leaky gut" and increased healthy anti-inflammatory markers in the body. Thus, diet can have a direct, positive effect on inflammatory bowel disease.

McCann, M.J., Johnston, S., Reilly, K., Men, X., Burgess, E.J., Perry, N.B., and Roy, N.C. "The Effect of Turmeric (Curcuma longa) Extract on the Functionality of the Solute Carrier Protein 22 A4 (SLC22A4) and Interleukin-10 (IL-10) Variants Associated with Inflammatory Bowel Disease." *Nutrients* 6, 10 (2014): 4178-90.

Obesity and Diabetes

Low-glycemic diets benefit patients with type 2 diabetes, heart disease, and some types of cancer. However, the effect of low-glycemic diets on weight loss and inflammation is not so clearly understood. Researchers concluded that a low-glycemic and low-calorie diet with moderate carbohydrates control inflammation, glucose, and insulin and promote weight loss better than a high-GI and low-fat diet.

Juanola-Falgarona, M., Salas-Salvado, J., Ibarrola-Jurado, N., Rabassa-Soler, A., Diaz-Lopez, A., Guasch-Ferre, M., Hernandez-Alonso, P., Balanza, R., and Bullo, M. "Effect of the Glycemic Index of the Diet on Weight Loss, Modulation of Satiety, Inflammation, and Other Metabolic Risk Factors: A Randomized Controlled Trial." *American Journal of Clinical Nutrition* 100, 1 (2014): 27-35.

Obesity

Recent studies have shown dietary polyphenols may help prevent obesity and obesity-related chronic diseases. The effect of polyphenols found in green tea, resveratrol, and curcumin on obesity and obesity-related inflammation was evaluated. Cellular studies showed that these polyphenols reduce viability of fat cells, suppress fat cell development, stimulate the breakdown of fats, and reduce inflammation. Animal studies strongly suggest that polyphenols described in this review have a pronounced effect on obesity as shown by lower body weight, fat mass, and triglycerides. Human studies are limited at this time, but randomized controlled trials are warranted to determine the potential benefit of polyphenols on obesity.

Wang, S., Moustaid-Moussa, N., Chen, L., Mo. H., Shastri, A., Su, R., Bapat, P., Kwun, I., and Shen, C.L. "Novel Insights of Dietary Polyphenols and Obesity." *Journal of Nutritional Biochemistry* 25, 1 (2014): 1-18.

Obesity

A diet high in slowly digested carbohydrates (whole grains, legumes, and other high-fiber foods) reduces chronic inflammation. This study found that among overweight and obese people, a low-glycemic-load diet reduced C-reactive protein (marker of inflammation associated with cancer and cardiovascular disease) by about 22 percent. This same type of diet increased a hormone (adiponectin) that protects against cancer and type 2 diabetes, liver disease, and cardiovascular disease. The important message from this study is that quality of carbohydrates matter in reducing chronic inflammation.

Neuhouser, M. L., Schwarz, Y., Wang, C., Breymeyer, K., Coronado, G., Wang, C.Y., Noar, Y., Song, X., and Lampe, K. "A Low-Glycemic Load Diet Reduces Serum C-Reactive Protein and Modestly Increases Adiponectin in Overweight and Obese Adults." *Journal of Nutrition* 142, 2 (2011): 369-74.

Rheumatoid Arthritis

This study explores the link between dietary fat consumption and inflammation. As our intake in unhealthy fat has increased, so has the rate of inflammatory diseases such as asthma, atherosclerosis, and autoimmune diseases such as rheumatoid arthritis. Over-activation of immune cells can trigger inflammatory diseases. Fats such as omega-3, best known for being found in fish, linseed oil, and sunflower oil, improve clinical outcomes for rheumatoid arthritis and maintain healthy immune responses.

Garvan Institute of Medical Research (December 1, 2006). "Healthy Bodies Help Fight Disease? Clues To How Diet Affects The Immune System." *ScienceDaily*. Retrieved June 16, 2015, from www.sciencedaily.com/releases/2006/11/061130191550.htm

Works Cited

American Urological Association. "Metabolic syndrome disorders, diet may boost prostate cancer risk." *Medical News Today*. June 20, 2015. http://www.medicalnewstoday.com/releases/277070.php

Berk, M., Williams, L., Jacka, F., O'Neil, A., Pasco, J., Moylan, S., Allen, N., Stuart, A., Hayley, A., Byrne, M., and Maes, M. "So Depression is an Inflammatory Disease, but Where Does the Inflammation Come From?" *BMC Medicine* 11, 200 (2013).

"Bifidobacteria: MedlinePlus Supplements." U.S. National Library of Medicine, Web. Accessed July 25, 2015. http://www.nlm.nih.gov/medlineplus/druginfo/natural/891.html.

Bredesen, D. "Reversal of Cognitive Decline: A Novel Therapeutic Program." *Aging* 6, 9 (2014): 707-717.

Casas, R., Sacanella, E. and Estruch, R. "The Immune Protective Effect of the Mediterranean Diet against Chronic Low-grade Inflammatory Diseases."*Endocrine, Metabolic & Immune Disorders— Drug Targets* 14, 4 (2014): 245-54.

Chassaing, B., Omry, K., Goodrich, J.K., Poole, A.C., Srinivasan, S., Ley, R.E., and Gerwitz, A.T. "Dietary Emulsifiers Impact the Mouse Gut Microbiota Promoting Colitis and Metabolic Syndrome." *Nature* 519, 7541 (2015): 92-96.

Dai, C., Zheng, C., Jiang, M., Ma, X. and Jiang, L. "Probiotics and Irritable Bowel Syndrome." *World Journal of Gastroenterology*: (2015). Web. Accessed July 25, 2015. http://www.ncbi.nlm.nih.gov/pmc/articles/PMC3785618/.

Degagné, E, Pandurangan, A, Bandhuvula, P, Kumar, A, Eltanawy, A., Zhang, M., Yoshinaga, Y., Nefedov, M., De Jong, P. J., Fong, L.G., Young, S.G.,Bittman, R., Ahmedi, Y., and Saba, J.D.. "Sphingosine-1-phosphate Lyase Downregulation Promotes Colon Carcinogenesis through STAT3-activated MicroRNAs." *Journal of Clinical Investigation* 124, 12 (2014): 5368-384.

DiGiorgio, R., Vlta, U., and Gibson, P.R. "Sensitivity to Wheat, Gluten and FODMAPs in IBS: Facts or Fiction?" National Center for Biotechnology Information. U.S. National Library of Medicine, n.d. Web. Accessed July 23, 2015.

Fasano, A. "Leaky Gut and Autoimmune Diseases." *Clinical Reviews in Allergy and Immunology* 42, 1 (2012): 71-78. http://link.springer.com/article/10.1007%2Fs12016-011-8291-x

Galland, L., "Diet and Inflammation". *Nutrition in Clinical Practice* 25, 6 (2010): 634-40.

Garvan Institute of Medical Research. (2006, December 1). "Healthy Bodies Help Fight Disease? Clues To How Diet Affects The Immune System." *ScienceDaily*. Retrieved June 16, 2015, from www.sciencedaily.com/releases/2006/11/061130191550.htm

Giugliano, D., Ceriello, A., and Esposito, K. "The Effects of Diet on Inflammation." *Journal of the American College of Cardiology* 48, 4 (2006): 677-685.

Halmos, E.P., Power, V.A., Shepherd, S.J., Gibson, P.R., and Muir, J.G. "A Diet Low in FODMAP'S Reduces Symptoms of Irritable Bowel Syndrome." Gut 146, 1 (2014): 67-75.

Hernández-Alonso, P., Salas-Salvadó, J., Baldrich-Mora, M., Juanola-Falgarona M., and Bulló, M. "Beneficial Effect of Pistachio Consumption on Glucose Metabolism, Insulin Resistance, Inflammation, and Related Metabolic Risk Markers: A Randomized Clinical Trial." *Diabetes Care* 37, 11 (2014): 3098-105.

Hu, Frank B. and Willett, Walter C. "Optimal Diets for Prevention of Coronary Heart Disease." *Journal of the American Medical Association* 288, 20 (2002): 2569.

Institute of Food Technologists (IFT). "What are Fructooligosaccharides and How Do They Provide Digestive, Immunity and Bone Health Benefits?" *ScienceDaily* 16 (July 2013). www.sciencedaily.com/releases/2013/07/130716115728.htm

Juanola-Falgarona, M., Salas-Salvado, J., Ibarrola-Jurado, N., Rabassa-Soler, A., Diaz-Lopez,

A., Guasch-Ferre, M., Hernandez-Alonso, P., Balanza, R., and Bullo, M. "Effect of the Glycemic Index of the Diet on Weight Loss, Modulation of Satiety, Inflammation, and Other Metabolic Risk Factors: A Randomized Controlled Trial." *American Journal of Clinical Nutrition* 100, 1 (2014): 27-35.

Konturek, P. C., Brzozowski, T. and Konturek, S.J. "Stress and the Gut: Pathophysiology, Clinical Consequences, Diagnostic Approach and Treatment Options." *Journal of Physiology and Pharmacology* 62, 6 (2011): 591-99.

Luckey, D., et al. "Bugs & Us: The Role of the Gut in Autoimmunity." *Journal of Medical Research* 138, 5 (2013): 732-743.

Manach, C., Scalbert, A., Morand, C., Remesy, C., and Jimenez, L. "Polyphenols: Food Sources and Bioavailability". *American Journal of Clinical Nutrition* 79, 5 (2004): 727-47.

Mao, B. D., Li, J., Zhao, X., Liu, Z., Gu, Y.Q., Chen, H., Zhang, A. and Chen, W. "In vitro Fermentation of Fructooligosaccharides with Human Gut Bacteria." *Food & Function* 6, 3 (2015): 947-54.

McCann, M.J., Johnston, S., Reilly, K., Men, X., Burgess, E.J., Perry, N.B., and Roy, N.C. "The Effect of Turmeric (Curcuma longa) Extract on the Functionality of the Solute Carrier Protein 22 A4 (SLC22A4) and Interleukin-10 (IL-10) Variants Associated with Inflammatory Bowel Disease." *Nutrients* 6, 10 (2014): 4178-4190.

Mente, A., DeKoning, L., Shannon, H.S., and Anand, S.S. "A Systematic Review of the Evidence Supporting a Causal Link Between Dietary Factors and Coronary Heart Disease." Archives of Internal Medicine 169, 7 (2009): 659-69.

Migliori, M., Panichi, V., De la Torre, R., Fitó, M., Covas, M., Bertelli, A., Muñoz-Aguayo, D., Scatena, A., Paoletti, S., and Ronco, C. "Anti-inflammatory Effect of White Wine in CKD Patients and Healthy Volunteers." *Blood Purification* 39, 1-3 (2015): 218-223.

Neuhouser, M. L., Schwarz, Y., Wang, C., Breymeyer, K., Coronado, G., Wang, C.Y., Noar, Y., Song, X., and Lampe, K. "A Low-Glycemic Load Diet Reduces Serum C-Reactive Protein and Modestly Increases Adiponectin in Overweight and Obese Adults." *Journal of Nutrition* 142, 2 (2011): 369-74.

Odenwald, M.A., and Turner, J.R. "Intestinal Permeability Defects: Is it Time to Treat?" *Clinical Gastroenterology and Hepatology* 11, 9 (2013): 1075-83.

Ohio State University. "Compound In Mediterranean Diet Makes Cancer Cells 'Mortal'." *Medical News Today*. MediLexicon, Intl., May 23, 2013. Web. Accessed June 16, 2015. http://www.medicalnewstoday.com/releases/260826.php

Rao, S. S., Yu, S., and Fedewa, A. "Systematic Review: Dietary Fibre and FODMAP-restricted Diet in the Management of Constipation and Irritable Bowel Syndrome." *Alimentary Pharmacology & Therapeutics* 41, 12 (2015): 1256-1270.

Sabater-Molina, M., E. Largue, F. Torrella, and S. Zamora. "Dietary Fructooligosaccharides and Potential Benefits on Health." *Journal of Physiology and Biochemistry* 65, 3 (2009): 315-28. National Center for Biotechnology Information. U.S. National Library of Medicine. Web. Accessed July 25, 2015. http://www.ncbi.nlm.nih.gov/pubmed/20119826.

Sleiman, D., Al-Badri, M.R., and Azar, S.T. "Effect of Mediterranean Diet in Diabetes Control and Cardiovascular Risk Modification: A Systematic Review." *Frontiers in Public Health* 3, 69 (2015).

Wang, S., Moustaid-Moussa, N., Chen, L., Mo. H., Shastri, A., Su, R., Bapat, P., Kwun, I., and Shen, C.L. "Novel Insights of Dietary Polyphenols and Obesity." *Journal of Nutritional Biochemistry* 25, 1 (2014): 1-18.

Zamora-Ros, R., Rabassa, M., Cherubini, A., Urpí Sardà, M., Bandinelli, S.; Ferrucci, L., Andrés Lacueva, C. "High concentrations of a urinary biomarker of polyphenol intake are associated with decreased mortality in older adults." *The Journal of Nutrition*, 143, 9 (2013): 1445-1450.

Zamora-Ros, R., Shivappa, N., Steck, S.E., Canzian, F., Landi, S., Alonso, M.H., Hébert, J.R., and Moreno, V. "Dietary Inflammatory Index and Inflammatory Gene Interactions in Relation to Colorectal Cancer Risk in the Bellvitge Colorectal Cancer Case-control Study." *Genes and Nutrition* 10. 1 (2015): 447.

About the Author

Jan Tilley, President and CEO of JTA Wellness, is a highly respected dietitian and national leader in nutrition counseling, wellness, and chronic disease management. Jan holds a MS in Nutrition and has over 20 years of experience in the food and nutrition industry. Over the past decade Jan has managed JTA Wellness, a highly successful private practice nutrition clinic in San Antonio, employing a team of professionals who work with patients using a science-based research approach to wellness. Jan is committed to helping at-risk clients develop a healthy lifestyle to combat chronic health issues.

Being a lover of healthy, delicious food, Jan has written numerous cookbooks and created hundreds of nutritious recipes that are available on her website at jtawellness.com. Her most recent cookbook, *Healthy Meals for Hurried Families*, is a collection of delicious family-favorite recipes that have been featured numerous times in print and other media. She has also written *Getting Your Second Wind*, a motivational guide outlining a path to wellness through physical activity and healthy eating. *Getting Your Second Wind* has encouraged thousands of individuals by giving them a fresh start toward creating a positive attitude and balanced lifestyle.

Eat Well to Be Well was birthed from Jan's passion for encouraging readers to take personal responsibility for their own health by giving them the tools to live their best life through the power of anti-inflammatory food.

In the spring of 2012, the Texas Academy of Nutrition and Dietetics awarded Jan the State Media Award, which honors an outstanding individual that has made a positive impact on the promotion of nutrition and dietetics through the media. The National Association of Women Business Owners awarded Jan the Entrepreneurial Spirit Award as a Mentor in 2014.